MW00510856

SIRT Food Diet + intermittent fasting

Contents

are for clarifying purposes only and are the owned by the owners themselves, not affiliated with this document.

Introduction

The Sirtfood Diet is a food lovers' diet. You cannot expect people to eat the way you do it for the long term. The Sirtfood Diet is turning all of that on its head.

The benefits are all from eating delicious food, and not from what you don't eat. The better food you consume, the greater the rewards you enjoy. It also encourages us to rekindle the lost relationships of enjoying mealtime. Whether it's being on a movie set, being on a music world tour, or managing a bustling home, the business you keep connecting with as a family, depends on what your daily life means. Meals are an event where all come together to enjoy the company of each other. That can be done easily with the Sirtfood Diet. Eat freely, without guilt. Knowing the food, you eat feeds on your wellbeing. The meal plans are realistic and easy to follow, while still delivering delicious meals. There's real satisfaction to see empty plates at the end of a meal and everyone is content. The word diet in this book's title can almost be a mishap. In the traditional sense this isn't a diet but a method of preparing for good. It's for anyone wanting to put their body in a healthier state and feel their best while still enjoying their life and food. It's for people who want to see big differences from small changes, and for those who want weight loss that can last without spending hours in the gym or starving. This book will change your mind set about a word' Diet' and it also covers all the questions that will come to your mind once you start reading it.

The sheer breadth of benefits experienced by people has been a revelation, all achieved by merely basing their diet on accessible and affordable foods that most people already enjoy eating. And that is all that the Sirtfood Diet needs. It's about extracting the advantages of daily products that we've always been meant to eat, but in the right quantities and formulations to give us the body composition and well-being that we all want so desperately, and that can finally change our lives.

It doesn't allow you to implement extreme calorie limits, nor does it involve grueling fitness regimens (although remaining generally active is a good thing, of course). And just a juicer is the only piece of equipment you'll require. However, unlike any other diet out there that focuses on what to eliminate, the Sirtfood Diet focuses on what to add.

I've experienced firsthand these astounding benefits, and so have my friends and family members. We've gone from saying we would never go on a diet to never eating any other way. Now it's your chance to experience and enjoy it too!

To sum it up, Sirtfood diet will help:

- To lose weight by burning fat but not muscles
- Burn fat from the stomach area
- Keep your body for long-term weight loss success
- To look and feel better
- Live a longer, healthier and perfect life

Chapter 1: Purpose of Sirtfood

What makes the Sirtfood Diet so powerful is their ability to switch to an ancient gene family that exists within each of us. The name for that gene family is sirtuin. Sirtuins are different as they orchestrate mechanisms deep inside our cells that involve things as essential as our capacity to burn fat, our sensitivity— or not — to disease, and eventually also our life span. The influence of sirtuins is so powerful that they are now referred to as "chief metabolic regulators." 1 Just what anyone who wishes to lose a few pounds and lead a long and healthy life would want to be in control.

Throughout recent years, sirtuins have, unsurprisingly, become the subject of intense scientific research. The first sirtuin was found in yeast back in 1984, and research only started in the course of the next three decades when it was reported that sirtuin activation enhances life span, first in yeast, and then up to mice. Why the excitement? Because the basic principles of cellular metabolism are almost identical from yeast to humans and everything in between. If you can manipulate something as tiny as budding yeast and see a benefit, then repeat it in higher organisms like mice, the potential for realizing the same interests in humans exists.

1.1 An Appetite for Fasting

That takes us to fast. Consistently, the lifelong restriction of food intake has been shown to extend the life expectancy of lower organisms and mammals. This extraordinary finding is the reason for the custom of caloric restriction among some individuals, where daily calorie consumption is lowered by about 20 to 30 percent, as well as its popularized offshoot, intermittent fasting, which has become a standard weight-loss method, made famous by the likes of the 5:2 diet, or Fast Method. While we're still looking for proof of improved survival for humans from these activities, there's confirmation of benefits for what we might term "health span"— chronic disease decreases, and fat starts to melt away.

But let's be real, no matter how significant the benefits, fasting week in, week out, is a grueling enterprise that most of us don't want to sign up for. Even if we do, most of us are not able to stick to this.

Besides this, there are risks to fasting, mainly if we practice it for a long time. We mentioned in the introduction the side effects of hunger, irritability, fatigue, muscle loss and slowdown in metabolism. Yet current fasting programs could also place us at risk of starvation, impacting our well-being due to a decreased intake of essential nutrients. Fasting systems are also entirely inappropriate for large proportions of the populace, such as infants, women during breastfeeding, and very likely older adults. Although fasting has clearly proven advantages, it's not the magic bullet we'd like it to be. It had to wonder, is this really the way God was meant to make us slim and healthy? There's certainly a better path out there.

Our breakthrough came when we discovered that our ancient sirtuin genes were activated by mediating the profound benefits of caloric restriction and fasting. It may be helpful to think of sirtuins as guards at the crossroads of energy status and survival to better understand this. There, what they do is react to pressures. If nutrition is in short supply, there is a rise in tension on our cells, just as we see in the caloric restriction. The sirtuins sensed this, which then switched on and transmitted a constellation of powerful signals that radically altered the behavior of cells. Sirtuins ramp up our metabolism, increase our muscle efficiency, switch on fat burning, decrease inflammation, and repair any damage in our cells. Sirtuins, in turn, make us better, leaner, and safer.

1.2 An Energy for Exercise

It's not just caloric restriction and fasting that activates sirtuins; exercise does too. Sirtuins orchestrate the profound benefits of exercise just as they do in fasting. Yet while we are urged to participate in routine, moderate exercise for its multitude of advantages, it is not the method by which we are expected to focus our efforts on weight-loss. Research shows that the human body has developed ways of adapting spontaneously and reducing the amount of energy that we spend while exercising, seven implying that in order for exercise to be a successful weight-loss strategy, we need to devote considerable time and effort. The grueling fitness plans are the way Nature intended us to maintain a healthy weight is even more questionable in the light of studies now showing that too much activity can be harmful— weakening our immune systems, harming the liver, and leading to an early death.

So far, we have discovered that the key to activating our sirtuin genes is if we want to lose weight and be healthy. Up until now, diet and meditation have been the two proven ways to achieve this.

Unfortunately, the amounts needed for successful weight loss come with their drawbacks, and for most of us, this is simply incompatible with how we live twenty-first century lives. Luckily, there is a newly discovered, ground-breaking way to activate our sirtuin genes in the best way possible: sirtfood. As we will know early, these are the wonderful foods which are especially rich in specific natural plant chemicals, which have the ability to communicate to our sirtuin genes and turn them on. Essentially, they mimic the results of diet and exercise, which offer impressive advantages by burning fat in doing so., muscle building, and health-boosting that were previously unattainable.

SUMMARY

- Each one of us has an ancient gene family called sirtuins.

- Master metabolic regulators are sirtuins that regulate our ability to burn fat and maintain a healthy state.

- Sirtuins serve as energy sensors inside our cells and are triggered upon identification of energy shortages.

- Both fasts and exercises activate our sirtuin genes but can be challenging to adhere to and may even have drawbacks.

- You will replicate the results of fasting and exercise by eating a diet high in Sirtfoods and create the body you like.

Chapter 2: Masters of Muscles

One surprising result from our pilot trial that puzzled us was that the participants' muscle mass did not drop; instead, it rose by just over 1 pound on average. While it was common to see weight loss on the scales of 7 pounds, we saw something fascinating happening too. The injuries on the levels initially appeared more disappointing than this for almost two-thirds of our participants, though still very impressive, with a weight loss of just over 5 pounds. But when tests were done on body composition, we were astonished. In these participants, muscle mass was not only maintained; it had increased. The total muscle benefit for this category was almost 2 pounds, adding 7 pounds to what is called a "muscle gain-based weight loss."

This was totally unexpected and in stark contrast to what is typically the case for diets for weight loss, where people lose some fat but also lose muscle. For any diet which limits calories, it's the classic trade-off: you kiss good-bye muscle as well as fat. This is not at all surprising when you consider that cells change from growth mode to survival mode as we rob the body of nutrition and will use the protein from the muscle as food.

2.1 What's Good about maintaining Muscles?

So, what's that big deal? Do you know? Firstly, that means you're going to look much better. Stripping away weight while maintaining muscle leads to a healthy, toned, and competitive body that is more attractive. And more specifically, you should remain good looking. The skeletal muscle is the main factor that accounts for the daily energy output of our body, which ensures the more muscle that you have, the more calories that you use, even when you rest. This helps support further weight loss and increases the likelihood of long-term success. As we now learn, weight loss with typical diet results from both fat loss and muscle loss, and thereby we see a marked decline in the metabolic rate. This induces the body to regain weight once more regular eating habits are resumed. But you burn more fat with a minimal drop in metabolic rate by holding your muscle mass with Sirtfoods. This provides the perfect basis for weight-loss success over the long term.

In addition, muscle mass and function are predictors of well-being and healthy aging, and maintaining the muscle prevents the development of chronic diseases such as diabetes and osteoporosis, as well as keeping us mobile into older age. Importantly, it also seems to make us happy, with scientists believing that even the way sirtuins retain muscle has implications for stress-related disorders, including depression reduction.

All in all, weight loss when maintaining the body is a biggie and an even more desirable outcome. It's a unique feature of the Sirtfood Diet, and we need to get back to the sirtuins, so their substantial impact on the muscle to better understand why.

2.2 Sirtuins and Muscles Mass

In the body, there is a family of genes that function as guardians of our muscle and, when under stress, avoid its breakdown: the sirtuins. SIRT is a potent Muscle Breakdown Inhibitor. As long as SIRT is activated, even when we are fasting, muscle breakdown is prevented, and we continue to burn fat for fuel.

But SIRT's benefits aren't ending with preserving muscle mass. The sirtuins work to increase our skeletal muscle mass. We need to delve into the exciting world of stem cells and illustrate how that process functions. Our muscle comprises a particular type of stem cell, which is called a satellite cell that regulates its development and regeneration. Satellite cells just sit there quietly most of the time, but they are activated when a muscle gets damaged or stressed. By things like weight training, this is how our muscles grow stronger. SIRT is essential for activating satellite cells, and without its activity, muscles are significantly smaller because they no longer have the capacity to develop or regenerate properly.6 However, by increasing SIRT activity, we give a boost to our satellite cells, which encourages muscle growth and recovery.

2.3 SirtFood Versus Fasting

This leads to a big question: if activation of the sirtuin increases muscle mass, why do we lose muscle when we fast? Fasting also stimulates our sirtuin genes, after all. And therein is one of fasting's big pitfalls.

Stay with us as we dig into the mechanics of this. Not all skeletal muscles are created equal to each other. We have two main types, named type-1 and type-2, conveniently. Type-1 tissue is used for movements of longer duration, while the type-2 muscle is used for short bursts of more intense activity. And here's where it gets intriguing: fasting only increases SIRT activity in type-1 muscle fibers, not type-2, So type-1 muscle fiber size is maintained and even noticeably increases when we fast. Sadly, in complete contrast to what happens in type-1 fibers during fasting, SIRT rapidly decreases in type-2 fibers. This means that fat burning slows down, and muscle breaks down to provide fuel, instead.

But fasting for the muscles is a double-edged sword, with our type-2 fibers taking a hit. Type-2 fibers form the bulk of our concept of muscle. So even though our type-1 fiber mass is growing, with fasting, we still see a substantial overall loss of muscle. If we were able to stop the breakup, it would not only make us look aesthetically healthy but also help to promote more loss of weight. And the way to do this is to combat the decrease in SIRT in muscle fiber type-2 that is caused by fasting.

Researchers at Harvard Medical School tested this in an elegant mice study. They showed that the signals for muscle breakdown were switched off by stimulating SIRT activity in type-2 fibers during fasting, and no muscle loss occurred. The researchers then went to one step forward and checked the effects of increased SIRT behavior on the muscle while feeding the mice instead of fasted, and found it triggered a very rapid growth of the muscle.

Within a week, muscle fibers with increased levels of SIRT activity showed an amazing weight gain of 20 percent.

These findings are very similar to the outcome of our Sirtfood Diet trial, though, in effect, our study has been milder. By increasing SIRT activity by eating a diet rich in sirtfoods, most participants had no muscle loss— and for many, it was only a moderate fast, muscle mass that increased.

2.4 Keeping Muscles Young

And that is not just the thickness of the body. SIRT's prolific effects on the muscle extend to the way it works too. As the muscle ages, it loses the ability to activate SIRT. This makes it less sensitive to exercise benefits and more vulnerable to free radicals and inflammation destruction, resulting in what is known as oxidative stress. Gradually muscles wither, become softer, and fatigue faster. But if we can increase SIRT activation, we can stop the decline associated with aging.

Indeed, by activating SIRT to stop the loss of muscle mass and function we usually see with aging, we see multiple related health benefits, including the halting of bone loss and prevention of increased chronic systemic inflammation (known as inflamaging), as well as improvements in mobility and overall quality of life. So, interestingly, the latest research indicates that the higher the polyphenol level (and thus sirtuin-activating nutrients) in older people's diets, the higher the security they enjoy against deteriorating physical performance with age.

Don't be fooled into thinking that those incentives extend only to the elderly, far from that. By the age of twenty-five, the signs of aging will begin, and the muscle gradually erodes, with 10 percent loss of muscle around age forty (although overall weight tends to increase) and a loss of 40 percent by age seventy. Yet there is growing evidence that the activation of our sirtuin genes will inhibit and reverse all of this.

Loss of muscle, development, and function: sirtuin behavior plays a crucial role in all of this. Stack it up, and it's no surprise that sirtuins were identified as master regulators of muscle growth in a recent review in the prestigious medical journal Nature, with growing sirtuin activation cited as one of the promising new avenues for combating muscle loss, thereby increasing the quality of life, as well as reducing disease and death.

Looking at the powerful effects our sirtuin genes can have on the muscles, our pilot trial's shock results no longer seemed so shocking. We started to realize that driving weight loss when feeding our muscles was achievable through a diet rich in Sirtfood.

But it's just the beginning. In the next chapter, we'll see Sirtfoods' benefits extending so much further, to all aspects of health and quality of life.

SUMMARY

- Amid weight loss, we found that people either retained or even gained muscle through the Sirtfood diet. This is because the sirtuins are chief muscle regulators.

- By activating sirtuins, muscle breakdown can be both prevented and muscle regeneration promoted.

- Triggering SIRT will help prevent the progressive muscle loss that we see with age.

- Activating your sirtuin genes will not only make you look leaner but will also help you stay healthier and function better as you age.

Chapter 3: Fighting Fat

One of the surprising results from our Sirtfood Diet pilot study wasn't just how much weight the participants lost, which was unusual enough— it was the amount of weight loss that fascinated us. What attracted our eye was the fact that a lot of people lost weight without missing any muscle. In reality, watching people gain muscle wasn't rare.

It left us with an inevitable conclusion: fat had merely melted away.

Achieving a substantial fat loss requires typically a tremendous effort, either significantly decreasing calories or participating in extraordinary exercise levels or both. Yet counter to that, our participants either retained or reduced their level of exercise and did not even report feel particularly hungry. In reality, some also refused to consume all of the food they had been supplied with.

Why is it even that possible? It is only when we understand what happens to our fat cells when there is elevated sirtuin production that we can begin to make sense of these remarkable results.

Mice that have been genetically engineered to have elevated SIRT rates are leaner and more metabolically involved, the sirtuin gene that causes fat loss. In comparison, mice who lack SIRT are more overweight and have more metabolic diseases. If we look at individuals, SIRT levels in obese people's body fat were found to be markedly lower than their healthy-weight equivalents. Those with elevated SIRT gene expression, on the other side, become leaner and more immune to weight gain. Scale all that together, and you begin to get a picture of how critical sirtuins are to decide how we stay lean or get overweight, and why you can produce these amazing results by increasing sirtuin activity. This is because we get advantages on multiple levels by sirtuins, beginning at the very heart of everything: the genes that regulate weight gain. To grasp this further, we need to delve deeper into what is occurring in our bodies, which is allowing us to gain some weight.

3.1 Busting Fat

We'll clarify this in terms of a drug-ring film in Hollywood. The streets flooded with narcotics is our body overflowing with fat. The drug pushers on the street corners are the source of the weight gain peddling responses in our heads.

But in fact, it's just the low-level losers. The real villain is behind it all, masterminding the entire operation, guiding any transaction that the peddlers make. This antagonist is referred to in our film as PPAR-π (peroxisome proliferator-activated receptor-ÿ). PPAR-ÿ orchestrates the mechanism of fat gain by clicking on the genes required to start synthesizing and storing fat. You will slash supply to avoid the accumulation of fat. Start PPAR-ÿ and you start fat gain successfully.

Meet our hero SIRT, who rises to push the enemy down. With the thief locked up safely, there's no one to pull strings, and the whole fat-gain enterprise crumbles. With PPAR-π's operation stopped, SIRT is turning its focus to "cleaning the streets." Not only is this achieved by shutting down fat development and storage, as we have seen, but it is changing our metabolism so that we continue to rid the body of excess fat. Like every successful crime-fighting character, SIRT has a sidekick, identified as PGC-1α, a central receptor in our cells. It actively encourages the formation of what is known as mitochondria. These are the tiny factories of energy that live inside each of our cells— they drive the body. The more we have the mitochondria, the more we can generate the oil. But as well as encouraging more mitochondria, PGC-1α also urges them to burn fat as the fuel of choice to make the electricity. So fat accumulation is prevented on the one side, and fat burning on the other decreases.

3.2 WAT OR BAT?

We have looked so far at the impact of SIRT on fat loss on a well-known fat type called white adipose tissue (WAT). This is the type of fat that weight gain coincides with. This specializes in preservation and growth, is persistent, and secretes a variety of inflammatory chemicals that prevent fat burning and promote more accumulation of fat, leaving us overweight and obese. That's why weight gain always begins gradually but can escalate so quickly.

But the sirtuin tale has another interesting twist, including a lesser-known type of fat, brown adipose tissue (BAT), which acts very differently. BAT is advantageous to us in complete contrast to white adipose tissue and needs to get used up. Brown adipose tissue helps us expend energy and has developed into mammals to allow them to dissipate large amounts of heat-shaped fat. This is regarded as a thermogenic influence and is essential to helping small mammals thrive in cold temperatures. Babies often contain considerable amounts of brown adipose tissue in humans, although it declines shortly after birth, leaving smaller amounts in adults.

This is where the activation of SIRT is doing something truly amazing. It turns on genes in our white adipose tissue so that it morphs and absorbs the characteristics of brown adipose tissue in what is considered a "browning effect." This suggests that our fat stores tend to function in a completely different way— instead of storing energy, they start mobilizing it for disposal. Sirtuin stimulation, as we can see, has an effective direct action on fat cells, allowing the fat to melt away. But there, it's not over.

The sirtuins also have a positive influence on the most critical weight control hormones. Activation of the sirtuin increases insulin production. It helps to reduce the insulin resistance— the failure of our cells to react to insulin adequately— which is heavily involved in weight gain. SIRT also stimulates our thyroid hormones ' release and operation, which play several standard functions in improving our metabolism and eventually, the pace we burn fat at.

3.3 Appetite Control

There was one aspect we couldn't get our minds around in our pilot study: the people didn't get hungry given a drop-in calorie. In reality, several people struggled to consume all of the food that was offered.

One of the significant advantages of the Sirtfood Diet is that without the need for a long-term calorie restriction, we can achieve great benefits. The very first week of diet is the process of hyper-success, where we pair mild fasting with an excess of strong Sirtfoods for a double blow to weight. So, we predicted sure signs of hunger here, as with all of the fasting regimens. But we've had virtually zero!

We found the answer, as we trawled through analysis. It's all thanks to the body's primary appetite-regulating hormone, leptin, called the "satiety hormone." As we feed, leptin decreases, signaling the hypothalamus inhibiting desire to a part of the brain. Conversely, leptin signaling to the mind declines as we fly, which makes us feel thirsty.

Leptin is so effective in controlling appetite that early expectations where it could be treated as a "magic bullet" for combating obesity. But that vision was broken by the fact that the metabolic disorder found in obesity causes leptin to avoid correctly functioning. Through obesity, the volume of leptin that can reach the brain is not only decreased, but the hypothalamus also becomes desensitized to its behavior. This is regarded as leptin resistance: there is leptin, but it doesn't work correctly anymore. Therefore, for many overweight individuals, the brain continues to think they are underfed even though they consume plenty, which triggers for them to continue to seek calories.

The consequence of this is that while the amount of leptin in the blood is necessary to control appetite, how much of it enters the brain and can have an effect on the hypothalamus is far more relevant. It is here that the Sirtfoods shine.

New evidence indicates that the nutrients present in Sirtfoods have unique advantages in overcoming leptin resistance. This is by both increasing leptin delivery to the brain and through the hypothalamus ' response to leptin behavior.

Going back to our original question: Why don't the Sirtfood Diet make people feel hungry? Given a decrease in blood leptin rates during the mild quick, which would usually raise motivation, incorporating Sirtfoods into the diet makes leptin signals more productive, leading to better control of appetite.

As we'll see later, Sirtfoods also has powerful effects on our taste centers, meaning we get a lot more pleasure and satisfaction from our food and therefore don't fall into the overeating trap to feel happy.

Sirtuins are expected to be a brand-new concept for even the most committed dietitians. But hitting the sirtuins, our metabolism's master regulators, is the foundation of any effective diet for weight loss. Tragically, the very existence of our modern society, with abundant food and sedentary lifestyles, creates a perfect storm to shut down our sirtuin operation, and we see all around us the effects of this.

The good thing is that we know what sirtuins are, how fat accumulation is managed, and how fat burning is encouraged, and most significantly, how to turn them on. And with this revolutionary breakthrough, the key to successful and lasting weight loss is now yours to bear.

SUMMARY

- Fat on Sirtfood Diet melts away. This is because sirtuins have the power to determine whether we stay thin or are getting fat.

- Activating SIRT inhibits PPAR-π, thereby preventing fat development and storage.

- Interestingly, triggering SIRT switches on PGC-1α, which allows our cells more fuel producers and enhances fat burning.

- On the Sirtfood Diet, you are unlikely to feel hungry because it tends to control the hunger in your brain.

Chapter 4: Well-Being Wonders

Society is getting fatter and sicker given all the incredible advances in modern medicine—70 percent of all fatalities are due to chronic illness, a truly shocking figure. Radical, and immediate, change is needed.

And as we've seen, all of this can begin to change. We will burn fat by stimulating our ancient sirtuin genes and create a leaner, stronger body. And with sirtuins at the center of our metabolism, our physiology master engineers, their significance reaches far beyond the structure of the body itself, to every aspect of our well-being.

4.1 What are Sirt Foods?

When we cut back on calories, this creates an energy shortage that activates what is known as the "skinny gene," triggering a raft of positive change. It puts the body in a kind of survival mode where fat is stopped from being stored, and healthy growth processes are put on hold. Alternatively, the body is shifting its focus to burning up its fat stores and putting on active housekeeping genes that rebuild and rejuvenate our cells, effectively giving them a spring clean. The upshot is weight loss and heightened disease resistance. But cutting calories, as many dieters know, comes at a cost.

Reducing energy consumption in the short term induces nausea, irritability, exhaustion, and lack of muscle. Long-term restriction on calories is causing our metabolism to stagnate. This is the collapse of all calorie-restrictive diets and paves the way for a piling back on the weight. For these reasons, 99 percent of dietitians are doomed to long-term failure.

All of this has prompted us to pose a big question: is it feasible to trigger our slim gene with all the great benefits they come and all those disadvantages without having to stick to an extreme calorie restriction?

Sirtfoods are especially rich in particular nutrients that can activate the same skinny genes in our bodies when we consume them as calorie restriction does. Those genes are called sirtuins. They first appeared in a landmark study in 2003, when researchers found resveratrol, a compound found in red-grape skin and red-wine, dramatically increased the lifetime of the petals. Incredibly, resveratrol had the same effect as calorie restriction on longevity, but this was achieved without reducing the energy intake. Studies have since shown that resveratrol has the potential to extend life in worms, fish, and even honeybees. Early-stage experiments from mice to humans indicate that resveratrol protects from the harmful effects of high-calorie, high-fat, and high-sugar diets; promotes healthy ageing by slowing age-related diseases and improves mobility. Essentially, the results of calorie restriction and activity have been proven to be imitation.

Red wine was dubbed as the first Sirtfood with its rich resveratrol material, describing the health benefits associated with its intake, and even why people who drink red wine get less weight. That is just the beginning of the Sirtfood tale, however.

The world of health research was at the cusp of something big with the discovery of resveratrol, and the pharmaceutical industry wasted no time jumping on board. Researchers have begun screening thousands of different chemicals for their capacity to activate our sirtuin genes. That revealed a number of natural plant compounds with significant sirtuin-activating properties, not just resveratrol. It was also found that a given food could contain a whole spectrum of these plant compounds, which could work together to both aid absorption and maximize the sirtuin-activating effect of that food. This had been one of the great resveratrol puzzles. Resveratrol experimenting scientists often needed to use far higher doses than we know when consumed as part of the red wine to provide a benefit. Nevertheless, unlike resveratrol, red wine contains a variety of other natural compounds for plants, including high amounts of piceatannol and quercetin, myricetin and epicatechin, each of which has been shown to activate our sirtuin genes individually and, more importantly, to function in combination. The dilemma for the pharmaceutical industry is that the next major breakthrough product cannot be sold as a vitamin or food category. So instead, they spent hundreds of millions of dollars in the expectation of uncovering a Shangri-la pill to create and conduct tests of organic compounds. Multiple studies of sirtuin-activating drugs for a multitude of chronic diseases are currently underway, and the first FDA-approved study to examine whether the drug would slow down ageing.

If we have learnt anything from history, it's that we shouldn't hold much hope for this pharmaceutical ambrosia, as tantalizing as that may seem. The medicine and wellness companies have continuously tried to emulate the effects of products and lifestyles by single supplements and medications.

And it has come up short again and again. Why wait ten more years for these so-called miracle medications to be approved, and the potential side effects they offer, because right now we have all the incredible benefits accessible through the food we eat at our fingertips?

So, while the pharmaceutical industry is chasing a drug-like magic bullet aggressively, we need to retrain our attention to dieting. At the same time, those efforts were underway, the landscape of nutritional research was also shifting, raising some big questions of its own. Red wine, on the one hand, were there other high-level foods of these different nutrients able to trigger our sirtuin genes? And if so, what effects did they have on triggering fat loss and combating disease?

4.2 All Fruits and Vegetables Are Not Created Equally

Researchers at Harvard University have conducted two of the most significant nutritional studies in US history since 1986: The Health Professionals Follow-Up Study, which examines men's dietary habits and health, and the Nurses' Health Study, which investigates the same for women. Building on this vast wealth of data, researchers explored the link between more than 124,000 people's dietary habits and changes in body weight over a twenty-four-year period ending in 2011.

They found something striking. Eating some plant foods staved off weight gain as part of a standard American diet, but eating others had no impact whatsoever. What were they different from each other? It all boiled down to whether there were different kinds of natural plant chemicals such as polyphenols that made the food beautiful. Almost all of us tend to put on weight when we mature, but the intake of higher quantities of polyphenols had a notable impact on avoiding this. Only certain types of polyphenols stood out when examined in greater detail as being useful in keeping people slim, the researchers found. The same groups of natural plant chemicals that the pharmaceutical industry was furiously trying to turn into a wonder pill for their ability to turn on our sirtuin genes were among those users.

The result was profound: When it comes to controlling our weight, not all plant foods (including fruits and vegetables) are equivalent. Alternatively, we need to start researching plant foods for their polyphenol material and then examine their ability to switch on our "skinny" sirtuin genes.

This is a radical idea that goes against the prevailing orthodoxy of our times. It's time to let go of the general blanket recommendations as part of a balanced diet that asks us to eat two cups of fruit and two and a half cups of vegetables a day. We only need to glance around to see how far that has had effects.

Something else became apparent with this shift in judging how plant foods are good for us. The many foods that supposedly health experts warned us off, such as chocolate, coffee, and tea, are so rich in sirtuin-activating polyphenols that they trump most fruits and vegetables out there. How many days are we grimacing when we chew our veggies because we are advised that this is the right thing to do, only to feel guilty if we even look at the sweet cookie during dinner? The ultimate irony is that cacao is one of the best foods that we might be consuming. The intake has now been shown to activate sirtuin genes, with multiple benefits for regulating body weight by burning fat, reducing appetite, and increasing muscle function. And that is before we take its multitude of other health benefits into account, more of which will come later.

In all, we have established twenty polyphenol-rich foods that have been shown to activate our sirtuin genes, and together these form the basis of the Sirtfood Diet. While the story began as the initial Sirtfood with red wine, we now know that these other nineteen foods equal or beat it for their sirtuin-activating polyphenol content. In addition to chocolate, these include other well-known and delicious products such as extra virgin olive oil, red onions, garlic, parsley, chilies, broccoli, bananas, walnuts, capers, bacon, green tea, and even coffee. While each food has impressive health credentials of its own, as we are about to see, when we combine these foods to make a whole diet, the real magic happens.

4.3 A Common Link Among all Other Diets

When we further researched, we learned that the most substantial concentrations of sirtfoods were contained in the diets of those with the lowest disease and obesity rates in the world — from the Kuna American Indians, who are resistant to high blood pressure and exhibit remarkably low rates of obesity, diabetes, cancer, and early death, thanks to a fantastically rich consumption of Sirtfood cocoa; to Okinawa, Japan.

But it's the diet that is the envy of the rest of the Western world, a traditional Mediterranean diet, where Sirtfoods stands out for its benefits. Obesity simply does not prevail here, and the exception is a chronic illness, not the norm. Extra virgin olive oil, wild leafy greens, almonds, fruit, red wine, seeds, and spices are all-powerful syrups, both appearing prominently in Mediterranean natural diets. Given the recent consensus that following a Mediterranean diet is more effective than counting calories for weight loss, and more effective than pharmaceutical drugs to stop the disease, the scientific world has been left in awe.

It takes us to the 2013 release of PREDIMED, a game-changing analysis of the Mediterranean Diet. It was performed on about 7,400 people at high risk of cardiovascular disease, and the results were positive that the study was effectively stopped early—after just five years. PREDIMED's premise was gorgeously simple. This asked what the difference between a Mediterranean-style diet augmented by either extra virgin olive oil or nuts (especially walnuts) and a more traditional modern-day diet would be. And what a difference.

The dietary change reduced the incidence of cardiovascular disease by about 30 percent, so drug companies can only dream of a result. With further follow-up, a 30 percent decrease in diabetes was also observed, along with significant drops in inflammation, changes in memory and brain health, and a massive 40 percent reduction in obesity, with substantial fat loss, particularly around the stomach area.

Yet researchers were initially unable to explain what these dramatic benefits produced. Neither the amounts of calories, fats, and sugars are eaten— the standard measures used to evaluate the food we eat— nor the levels of physical activity differentiated between the groups to explain the results. Something else had to get going.

The eureka moment then happened. Both extra virgin olive oil and walnuts are notable for their exceptional sirtuin-activating polyphenols content. Mostly, by adding these to a healthy Mediterranean diet in significant amounts, what the researchers unwittingly created was a super-rich Sirtfood diet, and they found it delivered terrific results.

So PREDIMED-analyzing researchers came up with a smart hypothesis. Unless actually, it is the polyphenols that count, they mused, then those who eat more of them would reap their combined benefits by living the longest. So, they were running the statistics, and the results were staggering. Those who consumed the highest polyphenol levels had 37 percent fewer deaths over just five years compared to those who ate the lowest. Intriguingly, this is double the mortality reduction that treatment with the most commonly prescribed blockbuster statin drugs is found to bring. Eventually, we had the reason for the mind-blowing benefits found in this test, and it was more effective than any existing drug.

The researchers also noticed something else unusual.

Although historically several studies have found that individual Sirtfoods impart remarkable health benefits, they have never been comprehensive enough to extend life potentially. The first such was PREDIMED. The difference was that they were looking at a food pattern rather than a single food. Different foods provide different polyphenols that activate sirtuin, which work in harmony to produce a much more powerful result than any single food can. This has left an irrepressible conclusion for us. Real wellness is not captured by a single nutrient or even a "wonderful meal." What you need is a full diet packed with a mix of synergistic Sirtfoods that all function. And that is what led to Sirtfood Diet being developed.

4.4 The Sirt Foods Empirical Study

Bit by bit, we've compiled all the observations from traditional cultures and the findings from major scientific studies, culminating in PREDIMED, one of the best dietary studies ever. But even PREDIMED's results came through chance as did many health breakthroughs. It never started to formulate and check a Sirtfood diet. Only later did science discover that this was indeed what PREDIMED had done.

This meant that the diet had not included many Sirtfoods that could have further increased its immense benefits.

In addition, all the research to date had identified the benefits for long-term weight management and disease reduction.

But we still didn't know how easily such effects could be recognized for body weight and well-being. We all want to protect our health in the future, but don't we want to look and feel right here and now?

To answer these questions, we wanted an experiment intentionally performed by the Sirtfood Diet that included all twenty of the most efficient SirtFoods with which we could collect earlier results measurements. So, we embarked on our pilot study.

Nestled in the middle of London, England, KX is one of the most coveted health and fitness facilities in Europe. That makes KX the perfect place to check the Sirtfood Diet's results is that it has its kitchen, which has provided us the chance not only to devise the diet but to bring it to life and evaluate it on the participants of the fitness center.

Our competences were obvious. Members would observe our built Sirtfood Diet for seven days in a row, and we would track their progress closely from start to finish, not only tracking their weight but also observing improvements in their body composition, which included testing how the diet influenced the fat and muscle levels in the body. Later, we added metabolic measures to see the diet's effects on blood sugar levels (glucose) and fats (such as triglycerides and cholesterol).

The first three days have been the most intense, with food intake limited to 1,000 calories a day. This is like a mild quick, which is necessary because the lower consumption of energy turns down signs of growth in the body and allows it to start clearing out old garbage from cells (a process known as autophagy) and kick-start fat burning. But unlike traditional fasting diets, this fast was gentle and short-lived, rendering it much more manageable, as shown by the exceptionally high adherence rate of 97.5 percent of the sample. We wanted to investigate the variations that were created by applying Sirtfoods to the usual drop associated with fasting diets. And they have been intense, as we were soon to find out.

Our primary objective was to make a big difference to the fat-burning results of this moderate calorie restriction by loading the Sirtfoods complete diet. This was done by basing the daily menu on three green beverages rich in Sirtfood, and one meal rich in Sirtfood.

At KX, calories were increased to 1,500 per day for the remaining four days of our study. Effectively this was only a rather small calorie deficit, but it turned down, and fat-burning signals turned up enough to hold development signals. Importantly, there was a jam-packed 1,500-calorie diet of Sirtfoods, comprising of two Sirtfood-rich green juices and two Sirtfood-rich meals per day.

4.5 The Results

The Sirtfood Diet was tested by forty, and thirty-nine members completed it at KX. Of those thirty-nine, two were obese in the trial, fifteen of them were overweight, and twenty-two had a healthy body mass index (BMI). The study was divided fairly even in gender, with twenty-one women and eighteen men. As participants of a health club, they were more inclined than the general population to participate and be conscious of healthy eating when they began.

The secret of many diets is to use a highly overweight and unhealthy sample of people to show the benefits, since at first, they lose weight the most and most drastically, effectively fluffing up the diet performance. Our rationale was the opposite: if with this relatively healthy population, we received good results, it would set the minimum benchmark of what could be accomplished.

The performance well exceeded our expectations, even healthy. The findings were clear and fantastic: an average weight reduction of 7 pounds in seven days after muscle growth is accounted for.

As if that wasn't inspiring enough, we've seen something else even more remarkable, which was the weight loss kind.

Typically, when people lose weight, they're going to lose some fat, but they're also going to lose some muscle— this is par for the diet course. We were amazed to discover the reverse. Our participants either kept their flesh or gained muscle. This is an infinitely more favorable type of weight loss, and a unique feature of the Sirtfood Diet, as we will find out later in the book.

No researcher struggled to see body composition changes. Yet note, without food deprivation or grueling fitness regimens, all this was done.

Here's what we found from our study

- Participants obtained spectacular and fast performance, dropping 7 pounds on average in seven days.

- Weight loss around the abdominal area was most noticeable.

- Muscle mass was either preserved or raised, rather than reduced.

- Rarely did the participants feel hungry.

- Participants felt a feeling of increased vitality and well-being.

- Participants reported having a better and healthier appearance.

4.6 Suirtins and The 70 Percent

Think of a condition you link with getting older and the likelihood of causing a loss of sirtuin involvement in the body. Sirtuin activation, for example, is excellent for heart health, protecting the muscle cells in the heart, and generally helping the heart muscle function better.[1] It also improves how our arteries work, helps us handle cholesterol more effectively, and protects against blockage of our arteries known as atherosclerosis.

As for diabetes? Activation of the sirtuin increases the amount of insulin that can be secreted and helps the bodywork more effectively. As it happens, metformin, one of the most common anti-diabetes medications, depends on SIRT for its beneficial effect.

Indeed, one pharmaceutical company is currently investigating the addition of natural sirtuin activators to diabetic metformin treatment, with results from animal studies showing a staggering 83% reduction in metformin dose required for the same effects.

As for the brain, sirtuins are again involved, with sirtuin activity found to be lower in patients with Alzheimer's. By contrast, activation of the sirtuin improves communication signals in the brain, enhances cognitive function, and reduces inflammation of the brain. This stops the accumulation of amyloid-β production and tau protein aggregation, two of the main damaging things we see happening in the brains of patients with Alzheimer's.

The next one is the teeth. Osteoblasts are a specific type of cell which is responsible for building new bone in our bodies. The more osteoblasts we get, the stronger our bones become. Activation of sirtuin not only stimulates the growth of osteoblast cells but also improves their survival. It allows the activation of sirtuin necessary for the protection of lifelong bones.

For sirtuin research, cancer has been a more controversial area. While a recent study shows that sirtuin activation helps suppress cancer tumors, scientists are only beginning to unravel this complex field. While there are so many other things to learn about this particular topic, as we shall see soon, those cultures that eat the most Sirtfoods have the lowest cancer rates.

Heart disease, arthritis, depression, osteoporosis, and most definitely cancer: this is an impressive list of diseases that can be avoided by sirtuin activation. It may come as no surprise to find out that cultures that already eat plenty of Sirtfoods as part of their traditional diets are experiencing longevity and well-being than most of us can hardly imagine, which you will hear more about very soon.

This leaves us with an exciting conclusion: only by adding the strongest sirtfoods in the world to your diet and having it a lifetime routine, you too can achieve this degree of well-being — and more — while you get the science you like.

SUMMARY

- For all the advances in modern science, we are getting fatter as a community.

- Seventy percent of all deaths are caused by chronic disease, with the vast majority having low sirtuin activity involved.

- Through triggering sirtuins, you can eliminate or forestall the Western world's most significant chronic diseases.

- By packing your diet full of Sirtfoods, you, too, can enjoy the same level of well-being as the healthiest and longest-living populations on the planet.

Chapter: 5 Sirt Foods

We've learned so far that sirtuins are an ancient gene family with the ability to help us burn fat, build muscle, and keep us super happy. It is well known that by caloric restriction, fasting, and exercise, sirtuins can be turned on, but there is another innovative way to achieve this: diet. We refer to the most active foods to activate sirtuins as Sirtfoods.

To understand the benefits of Sirtfoods, we need to learn about foods like fruits and vegetables very differently, and why they are perfect for us. Despite tons of evidence demonstrating that diets high in fruits, vegetables, and plant foods usually cut the risk of many chronic diseases, including the biggest killers, heart disease, and cancer, there is absolutely no doubt they do. This has been put down to their rich nutrient content, such as vitamins, minerals, and, of course, antioxidants, which is probably the greatest wellness buzzword of the last decade. But this is a very different story we are here to share.

The explanation Sirtfoods is so fantastic for you has nothing to do with the nutrients that we all know so well and hear about so much. Yes, they're all valuable things you need to get out of your diet, but with Sirtfoods there's something entirely different, and very unique. In reality, what if we turned that whole way of thinking on its ear and said that the explanation Sirtfoods is right for you is not that they nourish the body with essential nutrients, or provide antioxidants to mop up the damaging effects of free radicals, but quite the opposite: because they are full of weak toxins? This might sound crazy in an environment where almost every alleged "healthy food" is aggressively marketed focused on its antioxidant content. But it's a revolutionary idea, and one worth taking on.

5.1 What makes you stronger

Let's get back for a moment to the proven methods of triggering sirtuins: fasting and exercise. Evidence has shown consistently, as we have seen, that the allocation of dietary resources has significant effects for weight loss, wellbeing, and, quite likely, lifespan. Then there is fitness, with its numerous advantages for both body and mind, pointed out by the discovery that regular exercise slashes mortality rates dramatically. But what is the one thing they have in common?

The answer lies in: heat. All fasting and exercise cause the body to experience moderate stress that helps it to adjust by becoming stronger, more productive, and more durable. It is the reaction of the body to these slightly unpleasant stimuli— its adaptation— that, in the long run, should make us better, safer, and leaner. So, as we now learn, sirtuins orchestrate these highly beneficial modifications, which are turned on in the presence of these stressors, so spark a series of desirable changes in the body.

The technical term used to respond to those pressures is hormesis. It's the theory that if subjected to a low dose of a drug or stimulus that is otherwise harmful or fatal if administered at higher doses, you get a beneficial effect. Perhaps "things that don't kill you make you stronger," if you like. And that's just how fasting because exercising function. Hunger is fatal, so excessive exercise is prejudicial to safety. Such extreme forms of stress are inherently dangerous, but they have highly beneficial consequences, as well as diet and activity, to stay mild and controlled pressures.

5.2 Enter Polyphenols

So, here's where things get interesting. Many living organisms undergo hormesis, but the reality that this also involves plants is what has been highly undervalued until now. Although we would not typically think of plants as being the same as other living organisms, let alone humans, we do share similar responses in terms of how we respond to our environment on a chemical level.

As mind-blowing as that is, it makes perfect sense to think evolutionary about it, because all living things have adapted to encounter and deal with specific environmental pressures such as starvation, heat, lack of nutrition, and pathogens assault.

If it is hard for you to wrap your head around, get ready for that truly amazing part. Reactions to plant tension are, in general, more complex than ours. Think about it: if we're hungry and thirsty, we can go in search of food and drink; it's too humid, we're in the shade; we can escape under assault. By complete contrast, plants are stagnant, and as such, all the effects of these physiological pressures and challenges will survive. As a consequence, they have built a highly sophisticated stress-response system over the past billion years that humble anything we can boast about. The way they do this is to create a vast collection of natural plant chemicals — called polyphenols— that will help them to adjust to their climate and thrive. We also absorb certain polyphenol nutrients as we eat these products. Their influence is profound: they activate our inherent receptors to react to stress. Here we are talking about precisely the same directions that turn on to fasting and exercise: the sirtuins.

Piggybacking on the stress-response system of a plant in this fashion is regarded as xenohormesis for our gain. And the implications of that are game-changing. Nevertheless, because of their ability to turn on the same positive changes in our bodies, such as fat burning, that would be visible during fasting, these natural plant compounds are now referred to as reflective caloric constraints. And by supplying us with more sophisticated signaling compounds than we are generating ourselves, they cause effects that are comparable to anything that can be obtained by eating or exercising alone.

5.3 Sirt Foods

While all plants have these stress-response systems, only some have evolved to produce remarkable amounts of polyphenols that activate sirtuin. We are naming such plants, Sirtfoods. Their finding suggests there's now a revolutionary new way to trigger the sirtuin genes instead of austere fasting regimens or arduous exercise programs: consuming a rich diet in Sirtfoods. Best of all, this one involves putting Sirtfoods on your dish, not deleting it!

It's so beautifully simple and so quick it seems like a catch is required. But it is not. That is how nature intended us to feed rather than the rumbling stomach or calorie count of the modern diet. Many of you who have endured such hellish diets, where the initial weight reduction is temporary before the body protests, and the weight adds on again, would undoubtedly shudder at the thought of another false promise, another book advertising the infamous "d" term. Yet note this: the current dietary method is just 150 years old; Sirtfoods have been created by evolution about a billion years ago.

And with that, you're still curious to ask what Sirtfoods qualify for specific foods. So here are the top twenty Sirtfoods, without further ado.

SirtFoods	MAJOR SIRTUIN-ACTIVATING NUTRIENTS
Celery with leaves	apigenin
Chilies	luteolin
Parsley	apingenin, myrecitin
Garlic	myrecitin, agoene
Green Tea	epigallocatechin gallate
Kale	kaempferol, quercetin
red endive	luteolin
Red Onion	quercetin
Arugula	quercetin, kaempferol
Cocoa	epicatechin
Extra virgin olive oil	oleuropein, hydroxytyrosol
Walnuts	gallic acid
Buckwheat	rutin
Turmeric	curcumin
Soy	daidzein, formononetin
Strawberries	setin
Capers	kaempferol, quercetin
Dates	gallic acid, caffeic acid
Red wine	resveratrol, piceatannol
Coffee	caffeic acid

SUMMARY

- The belief that fruits, herbs, and plant foods are healthy for us has to be rethought entirely solely because they contain vitamins and antioxidants.

- We are good for us because we contain natural chemicals that put a little stress on our cells, just as fasting and exercise do.

- Plants also built a highly sophisticated stress-response system because they are stationary and created polyphenols to help them respond to their environment's challenges.

- As we consume these products, their polyphenols stimulate our mechanisms of the stress response — our sirtuin genes — emulating the results of caloric restriction and exercise.

- The product with the most sirtuin-activating activity is called Sirtfoods.

Chapter 6: Building a Diet That Works

We were doing something different with the Sirtfood Diet. We took the strongest Sirtfoods on the planet and woven them into a brand-new way of eating, the likes of which were never seen before. We picked the "best of the best" from the healthiest diets we have ever seen and built a world-beating diet from them.

The good news is; you don't immediately have to follow an Okinawan's traditional diet or eat like an Italian mamma. That on the Sirtfood Diet is not only utterly unrealistic but unnecessary. Sure, one thing you might be taken by from the Sirtfoods list is their familiarity. Although you may not consume all of the items on the menu at the moment, you are most definitely eating others. Then why don't you just lose weight already?

The answer is found as we explore the various elements that the most cutting-edge nutrition science indicates are needed to build a workable diet. It is about eating the right amount of Sirtfoods, range, and shape. It's about applying ample protein portions to the Sirtfood plates, and then enjoying your meals at the best time of day. And it's about the right to consume the authentic savory things you love in the amounts you want.

6.1 Hitting Your Quota

Most people just don't eat nearly enough Sirtfoods right now to evoke a strong fat-burning and health-boosting effect. Once researchers looked at the use of five primary nutrient-activating sirtuins (quercetin, myricetin, kaempferol, luteolin, and apigenin) in the US diet, human dietary intakes were found to be miserably 13 milligrams a day. Conversely, the average Japanese consumption was five times greater. Compare this with our Sirtfood Diet experiment, where everyday individuals ate hundreds of milligrams of sirtuin-activating nutrients.

What we are thinking about is a true diet change in which we raise by as much as fifty times our daily intake of sirtuin-activating nutrients. While that may sound overwhelming or unrealistic, it isn't really. Through taking all our top Sirtfoods and bringing them together in a way that is fully compatible with your busy life, you too can quickly and effectively reach the level of consumption required to enjoy all of the benefits.

6.2 Heard a Term 'Synergy'?

We believe it's better to eat a wide range of these wonder nutrients in the form of natural whole grains, where they coexist with the hundreds of other bio-active plant chemicals that act synergistically to improve our wellbeing. We think working for design is more comfortable, rather than against it. It is for this purpose that single nutrient supplements fail to show time and time again.

Take, for example, the classic nutrient resveratrol, which activates sirtuin. In supplement form, it is poorly absorbed; but in its natural food matrix of red wine, its bio availability (how much the body can use) is at least six times higher. Add to this the fact that red wine produces not only one but a whole host of sirtuin activating polyphenols that function together to offer health benefits, including piceatannol, quercetin, myricetin, and epicatechin. Or we could turn our attention from the turmeric to curcumin.

Curcumin is well established to be the critical sirtuin-activating nutrient in turmeric. Yet, research shows that whole turmeric has better PPAR-γ activity for fighting fat loss and is more effective at inhibiting cancer and reducing blood sugar levels than curcumin in isolation. It's not hard to see why isolating a single element in its entire food process is nowhere near as effective as eating it.

But what makes a dietary strategy different is when we start mixing several Sirtfoods. For starters, we are further enhancing the bio availability of resveratrol-containing foods by bringing in quercetin-rich Sirtfoods. Not only this, but they complement each other with their acts. Both are fat busters, but there are variations of how each of them is doing this. Resveratrol is beneficial in helping to kill current fat cells, while quercetin excels in avoiding the formation of new fat cells.6 In addition, all sides target fat, resulting in a more significant impact on the reduction of weight than just eating large amounts of a single food.

And this is a trend which we see again and again. Foods rich in sirtuin activator apigenine improve quercetin absorption from food and enhance its function. Quercetin, in effect, is synergistic with epigallocatechin gallate (EGCG) behavior. Yet EGCG's service with curcumin is synergistic. And so, it begins. Not only are specific whole foods more effective than single ingredients, but we tap into an entire tapestry of health benefits that nature has weaved — so intricate, so pure, it's impossible to try to beat it.

6.3 Juices and Food

Sirtfood Diet is a portion of both juices and whole foods. Here we are thinking about juices explicitly made from a juicer— blenders and smoothie makers (such as the NutriBullet) will not work. For many, this will seem counter intuitive, based on the fact that the fiber is lost when something is juiced. But this is just what we want for leafy greens.

Feed fiber includes what is called non-extractable polyphenols (or NEPPs). These are polyphenols, called sirtuin activators, which are bound to the fibrous portion of the food and only activated by our pleasant gut bacteria until broken down. We don't get the NEPPs by cutting the yarn, so miss out on their beauty. Importantly, though, the NEPP content varies dramatically based on the plant size. The NEPP quality in foods such as meat, cereals, and nuts are substantial and should be consumed whole (NEPPs contain over 50 percent of polyphenols in strawberries!). But for leafy vegetables, the active ingredients in the Sirtfood drink, they are much lower despite having a significant fiber content.

So, when it comes to leafy greens, by juicing them and eliminating the low-nutrient fiber we get full bang for our buck, so we can use even larger volumes and obtain a super concentrated hit of sirtuin-activating polyphenols.

There's another benefit of cutting the thread, too. Leafy greens comprise a form of fiber called insoluble fiber, which has a digestive scrubbing effect. But when we take too much of it, it can irritate and hurt our gut lining just like if we over-scrub stuff. This suggests that for many individuals, leafy green-packed smoothies can overwhelm fiber, possibly aggravating or even inducing IBS (irritable bowel syndrome) and hampering our nutrient absorption.

So, the bottom line is that we need to develop a lifestyle that blends all beverages and whole foods for maximum benefit to get the sirtuin genes going for dramatic weight loss and wellness.

6.4 Power of Protein

It's plants that bring the Sirt into the Sirtfood Diet. However, Sirtfood meals should always be rich in protein to gain maximum benefit. It has been shown that a building block of the dietary protein named leucine has additional benefits in activating SIRT to enhance fat burning and boost blood sugar control.

But leucine also has another part, and this is where it shines through its synergistic partnership with Sirtfoods. Leucine effectively induces anabolism (building things) in our cells, particularly in the muscle, which requires a great deal of energy and ensures that our energy factories (called mitochondria) have to work overtime. It induces a need for the Sirtfoods operation inside our cells. As you may remember, one of the effects of Sirtfoods is to promote the development of more mitochondria, to increase their performance, and to allow them to burn fat as fuel. Our bodies then need these to satisfy this extra demand for energy. The upshot is that we see a synergistic effect when mixing Sirtfoods with dietary protein that enhances sirtuin activation and ultimately gets you to burn fat to support muscle growth and better safety. For this purpose, the meals in the book are built to provide a large protein portion.

Oily fish is an exceptionally good protein alternative to supplement Sirtfoods' action because they are high in omega-3 fatty acids alongside their protein content. There is no way that you will have read a lot about the health benefits of oily fish and especially omega-3 fish oils. And now, recent research suggests that the advantages of omega-3 fats that come from enhancing the functioning of our sirtuin genes.

Over the past few years, many concerns have been raised about the adverse effects of protein-rich diets on wellbeing, and without Sirtfoods to counterbalance the protein, we can start to understand why. Leucine can be a knife with two-edges. We need Sirtfoods, as we have seen, to help our cells fulfill the metabolic demand that leucine imposes upon them. Without them, though, our mitochondria can become unstable, so high levels of leucine will promote obesity and insulin resistance, rather than improve health. Sirtfoods help not only hold the symptoms of leucine in check but also function effectively in our favor.

Speak of leucine as putting the foot on the weight loss and wellness generator, with Sirtfoods, the tool that ensures that the cell satisfies the increased demand. The engine blows, without the Sirtfoods.

Returning to questions about the health effects of protein rich diets, the missing piece of the puzzle is Sirtfoods. Usually, the US diet is protein-rich but requires Sirtfoods to counterbalance it, which makes it essential for Sirtfoods to become an integral part of how Americans live.

6.5 Try to Eat Early

The theory is the sooner, the better when it comes to food, preferably done feeding for the day by 7 p.m. for two significant reasons. Firstly, to harvest the Sirtfoods natural satiating power. Eating a meal that will leave you feeling full, happy, and energized as you go about your day is much more useful than spending the entire day exploring hungry just to feed and remain full while you sleep through the night.

But there's a second good reason to keep eating habits in line with your inner body clock. We also have an internal biological clock, called our circadian rhythm, which controls all of our normal body functions according to day time.

This affects, among other things, how the body handles the food we eat. Our clocks operate in synchrony, above all observing the signals of the sun's light-dark cycle. We're programmed as a diurnal species to be busy in the daytime rather than at night.

The body clock then allows us to handle food more efficiently during the day when it's bright, and we're supposed to be busy, and less so when it's night, where we're primed for rest and sleep instead.

The question is that many of us have "work clocks" and "social clocks," which are not aligned with the sun's slowing down. Sometimes after dark is the only option, some of us get to sleep. To some point, we will teach our body clock in synchronizing with different schedules, including "evening chronotypes" that want or need to be busy, eat and sleep later in the day. Life misaligned from the light-dark environmental process, therefore, comes at a cost.

Research shows that people with evening chronotype have decreased sensitivity to fat gain, muscle loss, and metabolic problems, as well as often suffering from poor sleep. That's just what we see in night shift workers, who have higher rates of obesity and metabolic disease, at least in part due to the impact of their late eating patterns.

The upshot is that when necessary, you're better off eating early in the day, preferably by 7 p.m. but what if that is simply not feasible? The good news is that sirtuins play a crucial part in synchronizing the body clock. Work has found that the polyphenols in Sirtfoods can modulate our body clocks and change circadian rhythm positively. This ensures the addition of Sirtfoods with your meal will mitigate the detrimental effects if you actually cannot avoid eating later on. Yes, one of the frequent comments we receive from Sirtfood Diet adherents is just how much their quality of sleep has increased, indicating the dominant influence on their circadian rhythm harmonization.

6.6 Embrace Eating

Let's give an idea. We just want you to do a very simple thing: don't think about a white bear.

What do you think? For a white bear. Why? For what? As we asked you not to think about it. Don't tell me that you're already there!

This was the trailblazing work conducted by psychology professor Daniel Wegner in 1987 that found that coerced repression of feelings creates a paradoxical and detrimental increase in how often we think about what we are attempting to suppress. So instead of removing it from our minds, the attempt generates a fixation with silenced thinking.

And as you've probably guessed, this trend doesn't just apply to white bears. The same thing happens when we are making heroes and limiting weight loss products.

Studies show that in general, we talk more often about them, rising the urge. It's eating away before we eat it! And now we are much more likely to binge with the diet disrupted and the heightened anxiety about the "forbidden" items we have experienced.

Now the physicists have clarified what's going on here. We all need to be fully autonomous. If we feel restricted, like being on a strict diet, this creates a negative atmosphere, which makes us feel uncomfortable. We get caught up in this misery, and we fight to get free. They protest by doing what we've been advised they shouldn't be doing and doing it a lot more than we would have at first. It happens to us all, even to the most self-controlled people.

It's not a matter of when but if. Researchers also agree that this is a fundamental explanation of why we can sustain diets and even see initial results but struggle to see long-term success.

So, does it really mean that there is no point in even trying to change our eating habits? Are we just doomed to fail? Yes, it implies that we need to create our own optimistic, ideal choice while making a transition to be successful. We already realize that it is not by dietary isolation but through dietary inclusion that we can do it. Instead of concentrating the attention on the disadvantages of what you shouldn't consume, instead, focus on the positive aspects of what you should eat. You avoid the social reaction by doing so. And the Sirtfood Diet's elegance is this. It's about what you bring in your food and not what you're throwing out. It's about consistency and not the amount of your diet.

And it's about you having to do it because you feel satisfied consuming great-tasting foods with the additional awareness that every taste offers a wealth of advantages.

Many diets represent a means to an end. They're about holding in there, trying to keep track of the "healthy dream." However, it rarely comes before the plan stalls, and it's never maintained, even if accomplished. There's a separate Sirtfood Diet. It's all about flying. Phase 1, which reduces calories, is held deliberately short and sweet to ensure positive effects are done before any adverse reaction happens. The emphasis then is entirely on Sirtfoods. And the desire to consume Sirtfoods isn't just motivated by a result of weight loss. But it is just as much if not more about appreciating and loving real food for a safe, active lifestyle.

What's more, once you enjoy Sirtfoods' unique benefits, from fulfilling your hunger to improving your quality of life, you'll see your preferences and tastes change. With the Sirtfood Diet, items that would have previously set off the chain of adverse reactions if you were told that you couldn't consume them would lose their appeal and diminish their influence on you. They become a small part of your diet, and they all met without a single white bear encounter.

SUMMARY

- The Sirtfood Diet draws on the planet's strongest sirtfoods and puts them together practically and straightforwardly to eat.

- It is necessary to eat Sirtfoods in the right amount, mixture, and ways to enjoy the synergistic effects of their sirtuin-activating compounds, in order to achieve optimal results for weight loss and wellbeing.

- Like our modern diets, Sirtfoods stimulates all of our taste receptors, ensuring that we get more satisfaction from our food and feel content sooner.

- By including other healthy ingredients, such as leucine-rich protein foods and oily fish, we further reinforce this to render the results of the Sirtfood Diet even more strong.

- The Sirtfood Diet is an inclusion diet — not isolation, rendering it the only form of diet that can offer weight-loss results over the long term.

Chapter 7: Top-Twenty Sirtfoods

Now that you know everything about Sirtfoods, why they're so powerful, and what it takes to create an effective diet that will deliver lasting results, it's time to get started. The next chapter marks the start of day one of the Sirtfood Diet. So, this is the perfect time to get acquainted with each of the top twenty Sirtfoods, which will soon become the staples of your daily diet.

Arugula

Arugula (also known as rocket, rucola, rugula, and roquette) has a colorful history in American food culture. A pungent green salad leaf with a distinctive peppery taste, it rapidly rose from humble roots to become an emblem of food snobbery in the United States as the source of many peasant dishes in the Mediterranean, thus contributing to the coining of the word arugulance.

But long before it was a salad leaf wielded in a war of class, arugula was known for its medical properties by the ancient Greeks and Romans. Commonly used as a diuretic and digestive aid, it earned its real popularity from its reputation for having strong aphrodisiac powers, so much so that the production of arugula was forbidden in monasteries in the Middle Ages, and the renowned Roman poet Virgil wrote that "the rocket excites the sexual desire of drowsy men." A mixture of kaempferol and quercetin is being studied as a topical product in addition to strong sirtuin-activating effects, as together, they moisturize and promote collagen synthesis in the skin. With those qualifications, it's time to drop the elitist tag and make this the leaf of preference for salad bases, where it beautifully combines with an extra virgin olive oil dressing, combining to create a powerful double act of Sirtfood.

Buckwheat

Buckwheat was one of Japan's earliest domesticated crops, and the story goes that when Buddhist monks made long trips into the mountains, they'd just bring a cooking pot and a buckwheat bag for food. Buckwheat is so nutritious that this was all they needed, and it fed them up for weeks. We're big fans of buckwheat too. Firstly, because it is one of a sirtuin activator's best-known sources, called rutin. But also, because it has advantages as a cover crop, improving soil quality and suppressing weed growth, making it a fantastic crop for environmentally sound and sustainable agriculture.

The explanation buckwheat is head and shoulders above other, more traditional grains is presumably because it's not a grain at all— it's a rhubarb-related fruit crop. Getting one of the highest protein contents of any plant, as well as being a Sirtfood powerhouse, allows it an unrivaled substitute to more widely used grains.

Moreover, it is as versatile as any grain, and being naturally gluten-free, it is a great choice for those intolerant to gluten.

Capers

In case you're not so familiar with capers, we're talking about those salty, dark green, pellet-like things on top of a pizza that you may only have had occasion to see. Yet inevitably, they are one of the most undervalued and overlooked foods out there. Intriguingly, they are the caper bush's flower buds, which grow abundantly in the Mediterranean before being picked and preserved by hand. Studies now reveal that capers possess important antimicrobial, antidiabetic, anti-inflammatory, immunomodulatory, and antiviral properties, and have a history of medicinal use in the Mediterranean and North African regions. It's hardly shocking when we find that they are filled with nutrients that trigger sirtuin.

Celery

For centuries, celery was around and revered — with leaves still adorning the ashes of the Egyptian pharaoh Tutankhamun who died about 1323 BCE. Early strains were very bitter, and celery was generally considered a medicinal plant, especially for cleansing and detoxification to prevent disease. This is especially interesting given that liver, kidney, and gut health are among the many promising benefits that science is now showing. In the seventeenth century, it was domesticated as a vegetable, and selective breeding reduced its strong bitter flavor in favor of sweeter varieties, thus establishing its place as a traditional salad vegetable. It is important to note when it comes to celery, that there are two types: blanched/yellow and Pascal / green. Blanching is a technique developed to reduce the characteristic bitter taste of the celery, which has been perceived to be too strong. This involves shading the celery before harvesting from sunlight, resulting in a paler color and a milder flavor. What a travesty that is, for blanching dumbs down the sirtuin-activating properties of celery as well as dumbing down the taste. Luckily, the tide is changing, and people are demanding true and distinct flavor, turning back to the greener option. Green celery is the sort that we suggest you use in both the green juices and dinners, with the core and leaves being the healthiest pieces.

Chilies

The chili has been an integral part of gastronomic experience worldwide for thousands of years. On one level, it's disconcerting that we'd be so enamored with it. The pungent fire, caused by a substance called capsaicin in chilies, is engineered as a method of plant protection to cause pain and dissuade pests from feasting on it, and we appreciate that. The food and our infatuation with it are almost magical.

Incredibly, one study showed that consuming chilies together even enhances human cooperation.1 So we know from a health perspective that their seductive fire is wonderful to stimulate our sirtuins so improve our metabolism. The culinary applications of the chili are also endless, making it an easy way to give a hefty Sirtfood boost to any dish.

At times when we appreciate that not everyone is a fan of hot or spicy food, we also hope that we can entice you to consider adding small amounts of chilies, especially in light of recent research showing that those eating spicy foods three or more times a week have a thirteen percent lower death rate compared to those eating them less than once a week.

The hotter the chili, the better its Sirtfood credentials, but be sensitive and stick with what suits your tastes. Serrano peppers are a great start-they tolerable for most people while packing heat. For more experienced heat seekers, we recommend searching for Thai chilies for maximum sirtuin-activating benefits. These can be harder to find in grocery stores but are often found in specialty markets in Asia. Go for deep-colored peppers, excluding those with a wrinkled and fuzzy feel.

Cocoa

Cocoa was considered a holy food and was usually reserved for the elite and the warriors, served at feasts to gain loyalty and duty. Indeed, there was such high regard for the cocoa bean that it was even used as a form of currency. It was normally served as a frothy beverage back then. But what could be a more delicious way to get our dietary quota of cacao than through chocolate?

Unfortunately, there's no count here for the diluted, refined, and highly sweetened milk chocolate we commonly munch. We're talking about chocolate with 85 percent solids of cocoa to earn its Sirtfood badge. But even then, aside from the percentage of cocoa, not every chocolate is created equal. To the acidity to give it a darker color, chocolate is often handled with an alkalizing agent (known as the Dutch process). Sadly, this process diminishes its sirtuin-activating flavanols massively, thereby seriously compromising its health-promoting quality. Fortunately, and unlike in many other countries, food labeling regulations in the United States require alkalized cocoa to be declared as such and labeled "alkali processed." We recommend avoiding these products, even if they boast a higher percentage of cocoa, and opting instead for those who have not undergone Dutch processing to reap the real benefits of cocoa.

Coffee

What's all that about Sirtfood Coffee? We're listening to you. We can assure you that this is no typo. Gone are the days when a twinge of remorse had to balance our love of coffee. The research is unambiguous: coffee is healthy bonafide food. Indeed, it is a real treasure trove of fantastic nutrients that activate sirtuin. And with more than half of Americans drinking coffee every day (to the tune of $40 billion a year!), coffee boasts the accolade of being America's number one source of polyphenols. The ultimate irony is that the one thing we were chastised by so many health "experts" for doing was, in fact, the best thing we were doing for our health each day. This is why coffee drinkers have significantly less diabetes, as well as lower rates of certain cancers and neurodegenerative diseases. As for that ultimate irony, rather than being a toxin, coffee protects our livers and makes them healthier! And on the other hand to the popular belief that coffee dehydrates the body, it is now well established not to be the case, with coffee (and tea) making a perfect contribution to the fluid intake of regular coffee drinkers. So, while we appreciate that coffee is not for everybody, and some people may be susceptible to the effects of caffeine, it's happy days for those who enjoy a cup of joe.

Extra Virgin Olive Oil

Olive oil is the most renowned of Mediterranean traditional diets. The olive tree is among the world's oldest-known planted plants, sometimes established as the "immortal vine." And since people began squeezing olives in stone mortars to collect them, its oil has been revered, almost 7,000 years ago. Hippocrates quoted it as a cure-all; now, a few millennia later, modern science unequivocally asserts its marvelous health benefits. There is now a rich scientific data showing that regular olive oil consumption is highly cardioprotective, as well as playing a role in reducing the risk of major modern-day diseases such as diabetes, certain cancers, and osteoporosis, and associated with increased longevity.

Garlic

Garlic has been considered one of Nature's wonder foods for thousands of years, with healing and rejuvenating powers. Egyptians feed pyramid workers with garlic to enhance their defenses, avoid various diseases, and improve their performance by their ability to prevent exhaustion. Garlic is a natural antibiotic and antifungal that is often used to help treat ulcers in the stomach.

Through facilitating the removal of body waste products, it can activate the lymphatic system to "detox." Besides being investigated for fat loss, it also packs a potent heart health punch, lowering cholesterol by about 10 percent and lowering blood pressure by 5 to 7 percent, as well as lowering blood and blood sugar stickiness. And if you are really concerned about the taste of garlic being off-putting, take note. When women were asked to assess a selection of men's body odors, it was judged that those men who consumed four or more garlic cloves a day had a much more attractive and pleasant smell. Researchers believe this is because it is considered to be a better signal for safety.

And there's always mints for fresher breath, of course!

Green Tea

Many will be acquainted with green tea, the toast of the Orient, and ever more common in the West. As the growing awareness of its health benefits, green tea intake is related to less obesity, heart disease, diabetes, and osteoporosis. The explanation it is believed that green tea is so healthy for us is primarily due to its rich content of a group of powerful plant compounds named catechins, the star of the show is a particular type of sirtuin-activating catechin known as epigallocatechin gallate (EGCG).

What's the fuss about matcha, though? We like to think of matcha on the steroids as normal green tea. In contrast to traditional green tea, which is prepared as an infusion, it is a special powdered green tea which is prepared by dissolving directly in water. The upshot of consuming matcha is that it contains dramatically higher levels of the sirtuin-activating compound EGCG than other green tea types. Zen priests describe matcha as the "ultimate mental and medical remedy that can make one's life more complete" if you are looking for further endorsement.

Kale

We are at heart cynics, so we are always skeptical about what drives the latest craze for superfood advertising. Is it science, or are its interests at stake? In recent years few foods have exploded as dramatically as kale on the health scene. Described as the "lean, green brassica queen" (referring to its cruciferous vegetable family), it has become the chic vegetable for which all health-lovers and foodies are gunning. Each October, there is even a National Day of the Kale. But you don't have to wait until then to show your kale pride: there are also T-shirts, with trendy slogans like "Powered by Kale" and "Highway to Kale." That's enough for us to set the alarm bells ringing.

We've done the research, filled with suspicions, and we have to admit that we conclude that kale deserves her pleasures (although we still don't recommend the T-shirts!). The reason we're pro-kale is that it boasts bumper amounts of the quercetin and kaempferol sirtuin-activating nutrients, making it a must-include in the Sirtfood Diet and the base of our green Sirtfood juice. What's so refreshing about kale is that kale is available everywhere, locally grown, and very affordable, unlike the usual exotic, hard-to-source, and exorbitantly priced so-called superfoods.

Medjool Dates

It may come as a surprise to include Medjool dates in a list of foods that stimulate weight loss and promote health — especially when we tell you that Medjool dates contain a staggering 66 percent sugar. Sugar doesn't have any sirtuin-activating properties at all; rather, it has well-established links to obesity, heart disease, and diabetes — just the opposite of what we're looking to achieve. But processed and replenished sugar is very different from sugar carried in a nature-borne vehicle balanced with sirtuin-activating polyphenols: the date Medjool.

Parsley

Parsley is something of a culinary conundrum. It so often appears in recipes, yet so often it's the green token guy. At best, we serve a couple of chopped sprigs and tossed as an afterthought on a meal, at worst a solitary sprig for decorative purposes only. This way, there on the plate, it is often always languishing even after we have finished eating. This culinary styling stems from its traditional use in ancient Rome as a garnish for eating after meals in order to refresh breath, rather than being part of the meal itself. And what a shame, because parsley is a fantastic food that packs a vibrant, refreshing taste full of character.

Taste aside, what makes parsley special is that it is an excellent source of the sirtuin-activating nutrient apigenin, a real boon since it is seldom found in other foods in significant quantities. In our brains, apigenin binds fascinatingly to the benzodiazepine receptors, helping us to relax and help us to sleep. Stack it all up, and its time we enjoyed parsley not as omnipresent food confetti, but as a food in its own right to reap the wonderful health benefits that it can bring.

Red Endive

Endive is a relatively new kid on the block in so far as vegetables go. The story has it that a Belgian farmer discovered endive in 1830, by accident. The farmer stored chicory roots in his cellar, and then used them as a type of coffee substitute, only to forget them. Upon his return, he discovered that white leaves had sprouted, which he found to be tender, crunchy, and rather delicious upon degustation. Endive is now grown all over the world, including the USA, and earns its Sirtfood badge thanks to its impressive sirtuin activator luteolin content. And besides the established sirtuin-activating benefits, luteolin consumption has become a promising approach to therapy to improve sociability in autistic children.

Note that its texture is crisp and a sweet flavor for those new to endive, accompanied by a gentle and pleasant bitterness. If you're ever stuck on how to increase endive in your diet, you can't lose by adding her leaves to a salad where her welcome, tart flavor adds the perfect bite to an extra virgin olive oil dressing based on zesty. Red is best, just like an onion, but the yellow variety can also be considered a Sirtfood. So while the red type may sometimes be more difficult to find, you should rest assured that yellow is an entirely appropriate substitute.

Red Onions

Since the period of our ancient ancestors, onions have been a dietary staple, being one of the first crops to be grown, around 5,000 years ago. With such a long history of use and such potent health-giving properties, many cultures that came before us have revered onions. They were held especially by the Egyptians as objects of worship, regarding their circle-within-a-circle structure as symbolic of eternal life. And the Greeks assumed that onions make competitors better. Athletes will eat their way through vast amounts of onions before the Olympic Games, also consuming the fruit! It's an incredible testimony to how valuable ancient dietary wisdom can be when we consider that onions earn their top twenty Sirtfood status because they're chock-full of the sirtuin-activating compound quercetin — the very compound that the sports science world has recently started actively researching and marketing to improve sports performance.

And why the red ones? Simply because they have the highest content of quercetin, although the standard yellow ones do not lag too far behind and are also a good inclusion.

Red Wine

Any list of the top twenty Sirtfoods would not be complete without the inclusion of the initial Sirtfood, red wine. The French paradox made headlines in the early 1990s, with it being discovered that despite the French appearing to do everything wrong when it came to health (smoking, lack of exercise, and rich food consumption), they had lower death rates from heart disease than countries like the United States. Physicians proposed the explanation for this was the copious amount of red wine drank. Danish researchers then published work in 1995 to show that low-to-moderate consumption of red wine reduced death rates. In contrast, similar levels of beer alcohol did not affect, and similar intakes of hard liquors increased death rates. Naturally, in 2003, the rich content of red wine from a bevy of sirtuin-activating nutrients was uncovered, and the rest, as they say, was made history.

But there is even more to the impressive resume in red wine. Red wine seems to be able to keep away from the common cold, with moderate wine drinkers having an incidence reduction of more than 40 percent. Research now also shows advantages for oral health and cavity protection. With average consumption, social bonding, and out-of-the-box thinking have also been shown to increase, that after-work drink among colleagues appears to have a basis in solid science to discuss work projects.

Soy

Soy products have a long history as an integral part of the diet of many countries in Asia-Pacific, such as China, Japan, and Korea. Researchers first turned on to soy after finding that high soy-consuming countries had significantly lower rates of certain cancers, particularly breast and prostate cancers. This is thought to be due to a special group of polyphenols in soybeans known as isoflavones, which may favorably change how estrogens work in the body, including daidzein and formononetin sirtuin-activators. Soy product consumption has also been linked to a reduction in the incidence or severity of a variety of conditions such as cardiovascular disease, symptoms of menopause, and bone loss.

Strawberries

In recent years, the fruit has become increasingly vilified, getting a bad rap in the growing fervor toward sugar. Fortunately, such a malignant reputation couldn't be more undeserved for berry-lovers. While all berries are powerhouses of nutrition, strawberries are earning their top twenty Sirtfood status due to their abundance of the fisetin sirtuin-activator. And now, studies support regular eating strawberries to promote healthy growth, keeping off Alzheimer's, obesity, diabetes, heart disease, so osteoporosis. As for their sugar content, a mere teaspoon of sugar per 31/2 ounces is very low.

Intriguingly, and inherently low in sugar itself, strawberries have pronounced effects on how the body handles carbohydrates. What researchers have found is that adding strawberries to carbohydrates reduces the demand for insulin, essentially turning the food into a sustained energy releaser. Yet new research also shows that eating strawberries in diabetes care has similar effects on drug therapy. William Butler, the great physician of the seventeenth century, wrote in praise of the strawberry: "Doubtless God could have made a better berry, but without a doubt, God never did." We can only agree.

61

Turmeric

Turmeric, a cousin of ginger, is the new kid in food trends on the block, with Google naming it the ingredient of the 2015 breakout star. Although we are only turning to it nowhere in the West, it has been appreciated for thousands of years in Asia, for both culinary and medical reasons. Incredibly, India is producing almost the entire world's turmeric supply, consuming 80 percent of it. In addition to the benefits of the "golden spice" we saw on pages 60–61, in Asia, turmeric is used to treat skin conditions like acne, psoriasis, dermatitis, and rash. Before Indian marriages, there is a ritual where the turmeric paste is added as a skincare treatment to the bride and groom but also to symbolize the warding off darkness.

One factor that prevents turmeric's potency is that its main sirtuin-activating compound, curcumin, is poorly absorbed by the body when we consume it. Research, however, shows that we can overcome this by cooking it in liquid, adding fat, and adding black pepper, all of which increase its absorption dramatically. This fits perfectly with traditional Indian cuisine, wherein curries and other hot dishes it is typically combined with ghee and black pepper, and yet again proves that science only catches up with the age-old wisdom of traditional eating methods.

Walnuts

Dating back to 7000 BCE, walnuts are the oldest known human-made tree food, originating in ancient Persia, where they were the preserve of royalty. Fast forward to the present day, and walnuts are a success story in the US. California is leading the way, with California's Central Valley famous for being the prime walnut-growing area. California walnuts provide the United States with 99 percent of commercial supply and staggering three-quarters worldwide walnut trade.

Walnuts lead the way as the number one nut for safety, according to the NuVal system, which ranks foods according to how nutritious they are and has been endorsed by the American College of Preventive Medicine. But what distinguishes walnuts for us is how they are ay in the face of conventional thinking: they are high in fat and calories, yet well-established to reduce weight and reduce the risk of metabolic diseases such as cardiovascular disease and diabetes. That is the power of activating the sirtuin.

The emerging research showing walnuts to be a powerful anti-aging food is less well known but equally intriguing. Evidence often refers to their advantages as a brain food with the ability to slow down brain ageing and reduce the risk of degenerative brain diseases, as well as reducing the deterioration of physical function with age.

Chapter 8: 7 Pounds in Seven days (Phase 1)

Hello to Sirtfood Diet, Step 1. This is the period of hyper-success, where you will take a massive move in creating a slimmer, leaner body. Follow our easy step-by-step directions and use the delicious recipes you'll find. We also have a meat-free version in addition to our regular seven-day schedule, which is suitable for vegetarians and vegans alike. Feel free to go along with whatever you want.

8.1 What to Expect

You'll enjoy the full benefits of our clinically proven strategy of dropping 7 pounds in seven days during Phase 1. Yet note that involves adding strength, so don't hang up simply with the percentages on the scales. Nor should you become used to measuring yourself every day. In reality, in the last few days of Phase 1, we often see the scales rising due to muscle growth, although waistlines continue to shrink. So, we want you to look at the charts, but not be controlled by them. Find out how you feel inside the mirror, if your clothes fit, or if you need to push a knot on your belt. These are all perfect measures of the underlying shifts in your body composition.

Be mindful of other improvements, too, such as wellbeing, energy levels, and how smooth the skin is. In a local pharmacy, you can even get tests of your general cardiovascular and metabolic wellbeing to see improvements in factors like your blood pressure, blood sugar levels, and blood fats like cholesterol and triglycerides. Also, weight loss aside, incorporating Sirtfoods into your diet is a big step in making your cells fitter and more disease prone, setting you up for an extraordinary balanced lifetime.

8.2 How to Follow Phase 1

We will lead you through the full seven-day program one day at a time to make Phase 1 as plain sailing as possible, including the lowdown on the Sirtfood green juice and easy-to-follow, delicious recipes every step of the way.

This phase of SirtFood Diet has two different stages:

Days 1 to 3 are the most important and you can eat up to a limit of 1000 calories every day during this time, consisting of:

- Three times SirtFood green juices
- One main course

Days 4 to 7 will see the daily intake of food rise to a maximum of 1,500 calories, composed of:

- Two times SirtFood green juices
- Two main courses

There are very few laws with which to obey the diet. Mostly, for lasting progress, it's about incorporating it into the lifestyle and around everyday life. But here are a few easy but big impact tips to get the best result:

1. Take a Good Juicer

Juicing is an essential aspect of the Sirtfood Diet, and a juicer is one of the best health-care purchases you can make. Although price should be the determining factor, certain juicers are more effective at extracting the juice from green leafy vegetables and herbs, with the Breville brand among the best juicers we've tested.

2. Start Preparation

One thing is clear from the multitude of feedback we've had: those who planned ahead of time were the most successful. Get to know the products and techniques, and stock up on what's essential. You'll be amazed at how natural the whole cycle is, with everything planned and ready.

3. Save your Important Time

When time is tight, dress cleverly. Meals can be made the previous night. Juices can be produced in bulk and stored in the refrigerator for up to three days (or longer in the freezer) until their sirtuin-activating nutrient levels begin to fall. Only shield it from light, and only add when you're able to eat it in the match.

4. Eat Early

Eating early in the day is healthier, and hopefully, meals and drinks should not be consumed later than 7 p.m. But the plan is primarily designed to fit the lifestyle, and late eaters always enjoy great benefits.

5. Space Out the Juices

These should be taken at least one hour before or two hours after a meal to maximize the digestion of the green juices and dispersed throughout the day, rather than making them very close together.

6. Eat till You Feel Satisfied

Sirtfood can have dramatic effects on appetite, and some individuals will be satisfied before their meals are over. Hear your body and feed until you're full, instead of forcing down all the calories. Because Okinawans have existed for a long time, it states, "Feed before 80 percent full."

7. Enjoy the Diet

Don't get caught up on the end goal but keep aware of the road instead. This lifestyle is about enjoying food in all its glory, for its health benefits but also for the fun and pleasure it offers. Research shows that we are far more likely to succeed if we maintain our eyes focused on the road rather than the final destination.

8.3 Drinks

As well as the recommended daily portions of green beverages, other drinks can be easy drinking in Phase 1. Non-calorie beverages, usually regular juice, black coffee, and green tea. If your usual tastes are for black or herbal teas, do not hesitate to include these too. Fruit juices and soft drinks are left behind. Alternatively, try adding a few sliced strawberries to still or sparkling water to make your Sirtfood-infused health drink, if you want to spice things up. Hold it for a few hours in the fridge, and you will have a surprisingly cooling option to soft drinks and juices.

One aspect you need to be mindful of is that we don't suggest abrupt, significant changes to your daily coffee use. Caffeine withdrawal symptoms can make you feel bad for a few days; similarly, significant increases may be painful for those especially sensitive to caffeine results. They also recommend drinking coffee without adding milk, because some researchers have found that adding milk will decrease the absorption of the beneficial sirtuin-activating nutrients. The same has been observed with green tea but incorporating any lemon juice increases the absorption of its sirtuin-activating nutrients.

Note that this is the period of hyper-success, and while you should be comforted by the knowledge that it is only for a week, you need to be a little more careful. We have alcohol for this week, in the form of red wine but only as a cooking component.

8.4 The SirtFoods Green Juices

The green juice is an essential part of the Sirtfood Diet's Phase 1 program. All the ingredients are strong Sirtfoods, and in every juice, you get a potent mixture of natural compounds like apigenin, kaempferol, luteolin, quercetin, and EGCG that function together to turn on your sirtuin genes and encourage fat loss. To that, we have attached lemon, as it has been shown that its natural acidity prevents, stabilizes, and improves the absorption of the sirtuin-activating nutrients. We added a touch of apple and ginger to taste too. But both of these are available. Nevertheless, several people find that they take the apple out entirely once they are used to the flavor of the fruit.

SirtFood Green Juices (SERVES 1)

- Two handfuls (about two and a half ounces) kale

- A handful (one ounce or 30g) arugula

- A small handful (about one-fourth ounce or 5g) parsley leaves

- Two to three large celery stalks (five and a half ounces or 150g), including leaves

- Half medium green apple

- Half - to One-inch (1 to 2.5 cm) piece of fresh ginger

- Juice of a half lemon

- Half teaspoon matcha powder*

*Days 1 to 3 of Phase 1: added only to the first two juices of the day

*Days 4 to 7 of Phase 1: added to both juices

Remember that while we weighted all the amounts precisely as described in our pilot experiment, our experience is that a handful of measures work exceptionally well. In reality, they are the best tailoring the number of nutrients to the body size of a person. More significant people tend to have more massive paws, and thus get a proportionally higher volume of Sirtfood nutrients to suit their body size and vice versa for smaller people.

- Bring together the greens (kale, arugula, and parsley), and blend them. We consider juicers may vary in their efficacy when juicing leafy vegetables, and you may need to rejuice the remains before going on to the other ingredients. The goal is to end up with around 2 ounces of material, or about 1/4 cup (50ml) of green juice.

- Now, blend the Celery, apple, and ginger.

- You should cut the lemon and also bring it through the juicer, but we find it much easier to push the lemon into the juice by hand. You should have about 1 cup (250ml) of juice in total by this point, perhaps somewhat more.

- It's only when you extract the juice and are ready to serve that you add the matcha. In a bowl, pour a tiny amount of juice, then add the matcha, and mix vigorously with a fork or whisk. In the first two beverages of the day, we only use matcha, because it includes small amounts of caffeine (the same quality as a regular teacup). When wasted late, it can keep you awake with those not used to it.

- After the matcha is resolved, add the juice that left. Give it a final blend, and the juice is ready to drink. Easy to top up with plain water, as you like.

> For Days 1 – 3, you can take the juices at different times of the day, and then you can take on a standard meal, eat it at a time that suits you (preferably eaten for lunch or dinner).

DAY 1

- Three times Sirtfood green juices

- One main course either;

Fried shrimps with Buckwheat noodles + one-fourth chocolate bar

Or

Miso and sesame glazed tofu with ginger and chili stir-fried greens + one-fourth chocolate bar

DAY 2

- Three times Sirtfood green juices

- One main course either;

Turkey with capers and parsley and spiced cauliflower + one-fourth chocolate bar

Or

Kale and red onion with buckwheat (vegan) + one-fourth chocolate bar

DAY 3

- Three times Sirtfood green juices

- One main course either;

Chicken breast piece with kale, red onion, and red salsa + one-fourth chocolate bar

Or

Harissa baked tofu with spiced cauliflower + one-fourth chocolate bar

> For Days 4-7, you can take the juices at different times of the day, and then you can take on a standard meal, eat it at a time that suits you (preferably eaten for breakfast/lunch or dinner). But as per your appetite, you can continue to add in half to three-fourth ounce (15g to 20g) dark chocolate, each day at your discretion.

DAY 4

- Two times Sirtfood green juices

- Two main courses either;

MEAL ONE: Sirt Muesli

MEAL TWO: Pan-fried Salmon fillet with caramelized endive, arugula and Celery leaves salad

Or

MEAL ONE: Sirt Muesli (vegan)

MEAL TWO: Tuscan bean stew (vegan)

DAY 5

- Two times Sirtfood green juices

- Two main courses either;

MEAL ONE: Strawberry buckwheat (vegan)

MEAL TWO: Buckwheat noodles in a miso broth with tofu, Celery, and kale (vegan)

Or

MEAL ONE: Strawberry buckwheat (vegan)

MEAL TWO: Marinated miso with stir-fried greens and sesame

DAY 6

- Two times Sirtfood green juices
- Two main courses either ;

MEAL ONE: Sirt super salad

MEAL TWO: Grilled beef with red wine, onion rings, garlic kale, and herb-roasted potatoes

Or

MEAL ONE: Lentil sirt super salad (vegan)

MEAL TWO: Bean mole with bakes potatoes (vegan)

DAY 7

- Two times Sirtfood green juices
- Two main courses either;

MEAL ONE: Sirtfood omelet

MEAL TWO: Chicken breast (baked) with parsley pesto and red onion salad

Or

MEAL ONE: Sirt super salad (vegan)

MEAL TWO: Roasted eggplant wedges with walnut and parsley pesto and red onion salad (vegan)

Chapter 9: Maintenance

Congratulations on completing Sirtfood Diet Step 1! You should already have excellent results of fat loss and not only appear slimmer and more toned but also feel revitalized and re-energized. Okay, now what?

Having seen these sometimes-incredible changes ourselves, we realize how much you're going to want to see much better results, not just retain all those advantages. Sirtfoods are, after all, designed to eat for life. The problem is how you adapt what you learned in Phase 1 into your regular dietary practice. That is precisely what inspired us to develop a fourteen-day maintenance plan designed to help you make the transition from Phase 1 to your more usual dietary regimen, thus helping to maintain and expand the benefits of the Sirtfood Diet further.

9.1 What to Expect

You should maintain the weight loss results through Phase 2 and continue to lose weight gradually. Also, the one striking thing we've seen with the Sirtfood Diet is that most or all of the weight people lose is from fat and that many put some muscle on. So, we would like to warn you again not to measure your success solely based on the numbers. Look in the mirror to see if you look leaner and more toned, see how well your clothes fit and lap up the compliments you'll get from others.

Note that just as weight loss occurs, the health benefits will increase. In implementing the fourteen-day maintenance plan, you are helping to lay the foundations for a lifelong health future.

9.2 How to Follow Phase 2

The key to success in this process is having your diet packed full of Sirtfoods. We've put together a seven-day meal schedule for you to adapt to make it as easy as possible, with tasty family-friendly meals, filled with Sirtfoods every day to the rafters. Now what you need to do is to implement Seven Day Program twice to fulfill Phase 2's fourteen days.

On each of fourteen days, your diet will consist of:

- Three times balanced sirtfood meals
- 1-time sirtfood green juice
- 1 – 2 times optional sirtfood snacks

Also, when you have to eat those, there are no strict laws. Be agile throughout every day and suit them. Two basic thumb-rules are:

- Take sirtfood green juice either in the morning or at least half an hour before breakfast.
- Try your best to take dinner by 7 PM.

9.3 Portion Sizes

In Phase 2, our attention is not on calorie counting. For the average person, this is not a practical approach or even a good one over the long term. Instead, we concentrate on healthy servings, really well-balanced meals, and most notably, filling up on Sirtfoods so that you can continue to benefit from their fat-burning and health-promoting impact.

We've even designed the meals in the plan to make them satiate, making you stay full for longer. This coupled with Sirtfoods' innate appetite-regulating power, ensures you're not going to spend the next 14 days feeling thirsty, but rather comfortably fulfilled, well-fed, and highly well-nourished.

Just like in Phase 1, try to listen and be driven by your appetite. When you prepare meals according to our guidelines and notice that you are easily full before you finish a meal, then stop eating is perfectly fine!

9.4 What to Drink

During Phase 2 you'll need to include one green juice every day. This is to keep you top with high Sirtfoods prices.

Just like in Phase 1, you will easily absorb other fluids in Phase 2. Our preferred beverages contain remaining plain water, bottled flavored water, coffee, and green tea. Whether black or white tea is your preference, feel free to enjoy it. The same goes for herbal teas. The best news is that during Phase 2, you will enjoy the occasional bottle of red wine. Due to its content of sirtuin-activating polyphenols, particularly resveratrol and piceatannol, red wine is a sirtfood that makes it the best choice of alcoholic beverage. However, with alcohol itself causing adverse effects on our fat cells, restraint is still safest, so we suggest restricting the drink to one glass of red wine with a meal for two to three days a week in Phase 2.

9.5 Returning to Three Meals

You enjoyed only one or two meals per day during Phase 1 and allowed you plenty of versatility when you eat your meals. As we are now back to a more normal routine and the well-tested practice of three meals a day, learning about breakfast is a good time.

Eating a good breakfast sets, us on for the day, raising our levels of energy and focus. Eating early holds our blood sugar and fat rates in balance, in terms of our metabolism. The breakfast is a good thing that is pointed out by a number of studies, usually showing that people who eat breakfast often are less prone to overweight.

The explanation for this is because of our internal clocks inside. Our bodies are asking us to feed early in expectation of when we will be most busy and need food. Yet, as many as a third of us will miss breakfasts on any given day. It's a classic symptom in our crazy modern life, and the feeling is there's simply not enough time to eat properly. But as you will see, with the nifty breakfasts we have laid out for you here, nothing could be further from the truth. Whether it's the Sirtfood smoothie that can be drunk on the go, the premade Sirt muesli, or the quick and easy Sirtfood scrambled eggs/tofu, finding those extra few minutes in the morning will reap dividends not only for your day but for your longer-term weight and health.

With Sirtfoods functioning to overcharge our energy levels, there's, even more, to learn from getting a hit from them early in the morning to continue your day. This is done not only by consuming a Sirtfood-rich meal but above all by including the green juice, which we suggest you have either first thing in the morning — at least thirty minutes before breakfast— or mid-morning. We get a lot of reports from our personal experience of people who first consume their green juice and don't feel hungry for a few hours afterward. If this is the impact it's having on you, taking a couple of hours until having breakfast is perfectly fine. Just don't miss this one. Instead, with a good breakfast, you should kick off your day, then wait two to three hours to have the green juice. Be versatile, and just go with anything that suits you.

9.6 Sirtfood Snacks

You should keep it when it comes to snacking or quit it. There is a long debate on about whether consuming regular, smaller meals is better for weight loss, or just keeping to three balanced meals a day. The fact is, that does not matter.

The way we've designed the maintenance menu for you means you're going to eat three well-balanced Sirtfood-rich meals a day, and you may notice that you don't need a snack. But maybe you've been busy with the kids in the classroom, working out or dashing about and need something to take you into the next meal. And if that "little something" is going to give you a whammy of Sirtfood nutrients and taste delicious, then it's happy days. This is why we created our "Sirtfood bites." These smart little snacks are a genuinely guilt-free treat made entirely from Sirtfoods: dates, walnuts, cocoa, extra virgin olive oil, and turmeric. We recommend eating one, or a maximum of two, per day for the days when you require them.

9.7 Sirtifying Your Meal

We saw that the only consistent diets are those of participation, not exclusion. Yet real success goes beyond this— the diet has to be consistent with living in modern days. Whether it's the ease of meeting the demands of our hectic lives or fitting in with our position at dinner parties as to the bon vivant, the way we eat should be trouble-free. You will appreciate your svelte body and beautiful smile, rather than thinking about the demands and limitations of kooky products.

What makes Sirtfoods so great is that they are available, common, and simple to include in your diet. Below, when you bridge the gap between step 1 and daily feeding, you can lay the foundations for a modern, better lifelong eating strategy.

The key principle is what we term the meals "Sirtifying." This is where we take popular meals, including many traditional classics, and we retain all the great taste with some smart modifications and easy Sirtfood inclusions but attach a lot of goodness to that. You'll see just how quickly this is done in Phase 2.

Highlights include our tasty smoothie Sirtfood for the ultimate on-the-go breakfast in a time-consuming environment and the easy turn from wheat to buckwheat to add extra flavor and zip to the much-loved pasta comfort food. While classic, famous dishes such as chili con carne and curry don't even need much improvement, with Sirtfood bonanzas providing traditional recipes. Yet who has said that fast food means bad health? If you prepare something yourself, we mix the true vivid tastes of a pizza and through the shame. There's no need to say goodbye to indulgence yet, as our smothered pancakes with berries and dark chocolate sauce have demonstrated. It's not even a treat, it's breakfast, and for you it's perfect. Simple changes: you keep eating the things that you enjoy when maintaining healthy weight and well-being. And that is Sirtfoods, the culinary movement.

9.8 Fourteen-Day Meal Plan

Beyond our standard plan, we also have a meat-free version which is suitable for vegetarians as well as vegans. You can also mix it with whatever you want.

Each day you will consume

- Three times balanced sirtfood meals
- 1-time sirtfood green juice
- 1 – 2 times optional sirtfood snacks

BREAKFAST

Days	Breakfast
Day 1 & Day 8	Sirtfood Smoothie
Day 2 & Day 9	Sirt Muesli
Day 3 & Day 10	Yogurt with mixed berries, chopped walnuts, and dark chocolate OR coconut yogurt with mixed berries, chopped walnuts, and dark chocolate*
Day 4 & Day 11	Spiced scrambled egg
Day 5 & Day 12	Sirtfood smoothie
Day 6 & Day 13	: Buckwheat pancakes with strawberries, chocolate sauce, and crushed walnuts OR coconut yogurt with mixed berries, chopped walnuts, and dark chocolate
Day 7 & Day 14	Sirtfood Omelet or Sirt muesli

LUNCH & DINNER

Lunch	Dinner
1. Chicken Sirt super salad	Asian shrimp stir-fry with buckwheat noodles
2. Waldorf salad	Tuscan bean stew
3. Stuffed whole-wheat pita	Butternut squash and date tagine with buckwheat
4. Butter bean and miso dip with celery sticks and oatcakes	Butternut squash and date tagine with buckwheat
5. Tuna Sirt super salad	Chicken and kale curry with Bombay potatoes
6. Stuffed whole-wheat pita	Kale and red onion dal with buckwheat
7. Strawberry buckwheat tabbouleh	Sirt chili con carne
8. Strawberry buckwheat tabbouleh	Kidney bean mole with baked potatoes

9. Waldorf salad	Smoked salmon pasta with chili and arugula
10. Buckwheat pasta salad	Harissa baked tofu with cauli
11. Tofu and shiitake mushroom soup	Sirtfood pizza
12. Tofu and shiitake	Mushroom soup
13. Lentil Sirt super salad	Baked chicken breast with walnut and parsley pesto and red onion salad
14. Lentil Sirt super salad	Miso and sesame glazed tofu with ginger and chill stir-fried greens

Chapter 10: Sirtfoods for Life

Congratulations, all stages of the Sirtfood Diet have now finished! Just let's take stock of what you have achieved. You've entered the hyper-success process, achieving weight loss in the area of 7 pounds, which probably includes an attractive increase in muscle. You also maintained your weight loss throughout the fourteen-day maintenance phase and further strengthened the body composition. Perhaps notably, you have marked the beginning of your transformation of wellness. You took a stand against the tide of ill health, which strikes so often as we get older. The life you have decided for yourself is enhanced strength, productivity, and health.

By now, you'll be familiar with the top twenty Sirtfoods, and you've gained a sense of how powerful they are. Not only that, you'll probably have become quite good at including them in your diet and loving them. For the sustained weight loss and health, they offer, these items must stay a prominent feature in your everyday eating regimen. But still, they're just twenty foods, and after all, the spice of life is variety. What next, then? We'll give you the blueprint for lifelong health in this chapter.

It's about getting your body in perfect balance with a diet that's suitable and sustainable for everyone and providing all the nutrients we need that enhance our health. It's about keeping on reaping the Sirtfood Diet's weight-loss rewards using the very best foods nature has to offer.

10.1 Some other Sirtfoods

We've seen why Sirtfoods are so beneficial: certain plants have sophisticated stress-response mechanisms that generate compounds that trigger sirtuins— the same fasting and exercise-activated fat-burning and durability mechanism in the body. The greater the quantity of these compounds generated by plants in response to stress, the greater the value we derive from their feeding. Our list of the top twenty Sirtfoods is made up of the foods that stand out because they are particularly packed full of these compounds, and hence the foods that have the most exceptional ability to impact body composition and wellbeing. But foods ' sirtuin-activating results aren't a concept of all or nothing. There are many other plants out there that produce moderate levels of sirtuin-activating nutrients, and by eating these liberally, we encourage you to expand the variety and diversity of your diet. The Sirtfood Diet is all about inclusion, and the greater the range of sirtuin-activating items that can be integrated into the diet. Especially if that means you will obtain from your meals even more of your favorite foods to increase pleasure and enjoyment.

Let's use the workout comparison. The top twenty Sirtfoods are the (much more pleasurable) equivalent of sweating it out at the gym, with Phase 1 being the "boot camp." By contrast, eating those other foods with more moderate levels of sirtuin-activating nutrients is like reaping the rewards of going out for a good walk. Contrast that to the typical diet that has a nutritional value equal to sitting all day on the couch watching Television. Yeah, sweating it out in the gym is fine, but if that is all you do, you will quickly get fed up with it. The walk should also be welcomed, especially if it means that you don't just choose to sit on the sofa.

For e.g., in our top twenty Sirtfoods, we have included strawberries because they are the most prominent source of the sirtuin activator fisetin. Yet if we look more broadly at berries as a food group, we find that they have metabolic health benefits as well as healthy ageing. Reviewing their nutritional content, we note that other berries such as blackberries, black currants, blueberries, and raspberries also have significant amounts of nutrients that cause sirtuins.

The same holds with nuts. Notwithstanding their calorific material, nuts are so effective that they promote weight loss and help shift inches from the waist. This is in addition to cutting chronic disease risk. Though walnuts are our champion nut, nutrients that trigger sirtuin can also be found in chestnuts, pecans, pistachios, and even peanuts.

Instead, we turn our attention to food. Throughout recent years there has been in several areas an increasing aversion to grains. Studies, however, link whole grain consumption with decreased inflammation, diabetes, heart disease, and cancer. Although they do not equal the pseudo-grain buckwheat Sirtfood qualifications, we do see the existence of substantial sirtuin-activating nutrients in other whole grains. And needless to say, their sirtuin-activating nutrient quality is decimated when whole grains are converted into refined "clean" forms. Such modified models are quite dangerous groups and are interested in a number of state-of-the-art health problems. We're not saying you can never eat them, but instead, you're going to be much better off sticking to the whole-grain version whenever possible.

With the likes of goji berries and chia seeds possessing Sirtfood powers, also notorious "superfoods" get on the bandwagon. That is most likely the unwitting reason for the health benefits they have observed. While it does imply that they are healthy for us to consume, we do know that there are easier, more available, and better options out there, so don't feel compelled to get on that specific bandwagon! We see the same trend across a lot of food categories. Unsurprisingly, the foods that research has developed are usually good for us, and we should be consuming more of them. Below we mentioned about forty foods that we discovered have Sirtfood properties too. We actively encourage you to include these foods to maintain and continue your weight loss and wellbeing as you expand your diet repertoire.

Vegetables

- artichokes
- asparagus
- broccoli
- frisée
- green beans
- shallots
- watercress
- white onions
- yellow endive

Fruits

- apples
- blackberries
- black currants
- black plums
- cranberries
- goji berries
- kumquats
- raspberries
- red grapes

Nuts and seeds

- chestnuts
- chia seeds
- peanuts
- pecan nuts
- pistachio nuts
- sunflower seeds

Grains and pseudo-grains

- popcorn
- quinoa
- whole-wheat flour

Beans

- fava beans
- white beans (e.g., cannellini or navy)

Herbs and spices

- chives
- cinnamon
- dill (fresh and dried)
- dried oregano
- dried sage
- ginger
- peppermint (fresh and dried)
- thyme (fresh and dried)

Beverages
- black tea
- white tea

10.2 Power of Protein

A high protein diet is one of the most popular diets of the last few years. Higher protein intake while dieting has been shown to encourage satiety, sustain metabolism, and reduce muscle mass loss. But it's when they pair Sirtfoods with protein that things get brought to a whole new level. Protein is, as you may remember, a necessary addition in a diet based on Sirtfood to gain maximum benefits. Protein consists of amino acids, and it is a particular amino acid, leucine, which effectively complements Sirtfoods ' behavior, strengthening their effects. This is done primarily by changing our cellular environment so that our diet's sirtuin-activating nutrients work much more effectively. It ensures we get the best result from a Sirtfood-rich meal, which is paired with protein-based in leucine. Leucine's main dietary sources contain red meat, pork, fruit, vegetables, milk, and dairy products.

10.3 Animal Based-Protein

Animal products have been implicated in recent years as a contributing cause of many Western diseases, especially cancer. If that is the case, eating them with Sirtfoods may not sound like such a bright idea. Here's our lowdown to lay that to rest.

One of the significant concerns regarding milk is that it is not just a simple food but a highly sophisticated signaling mechanism to cause rapid offspring body production. Although this has a cherished meaning in early life, it may not be so common in adult life. Persistent and hyper activating the primary growth signal now correlated with ageing and the progression of age-related disorders such as obesity, type 2 diabetes, cancer, and neurodegenerative diseases. Notwithstanding the intricacies of this signaling system being a relatively new area of research and thus still very much an uncertain and theoretical possibility, this does explain why people might shy away from dairy products. However, the study points to one thing: if we add Sirtfoods to a dairy-containing diet, they inhibit mTOR's inappropriate effects on our cells, rescind this risk, making Sirtfoods a must-include with a dairy-based diet.

Generally, there are mixed reviews of the association between dairy and cancer. If we stack up all the study, mild dairy consumption is perfectly fine in the sense of a Sirtfood-rich diet and can deliver several useful nutrients to supplement Sirtfoods.

Poultry is ok when it comes to meat and cancer risk, but red and fried meats are much more suspect. Although data concerning them in breast and prostate cancer on the field is pretty thin, there is a legitimate concern that red and processed meat eating plays a role in intestinal cancer. Processed meat, such as sausages tends to be the worst perpetrator. Although there is no need to take it off the table, it should be included in just small amounts, rather than being a constant.

The good news for red meat is that research shows that cooking it with Sirtfoods rescues the risk of cancer, whether it's making a marinade with herbs, seasoning, and extra virgin olive oil; frying the beef with onions, or simply adding a nice cup of green tea to the meal or indulging in dark chocolate after dinner.

These all pack a punch from Sirtfood, which helps to neutralize the harmful effects of red meat. While we're all out to have the steak and consume it, don't go crazy. Red meat consumption is best kept at around 1 pound (500 g) per week (cooked weight), roughly equivalent to 1.5 pounds (700 to 750 g) fresh.

The link between egg consumption and cancer risk has not been investigated as extensively as meat and dairy products have, but there seems little cause for concern in this regard. Which eggs have been active in inducing is heart disease, instead? This is because they constitute a significant dietary cholesterol source. Thus, we are advised to restrict the use of eggs. Further countries, including Nepal, benefit interestingly. Who is right, then? The reason for siding with the latter is compelling. There is no linked routine egg intake with any increased risk of coronary heart disease or stroke. Although specific genetic disorders that involve a decreased consumption of dietary cholesterol, this limitation is not appropriate for the general population.

10.4 The Power of Three

The omega-3 long-chain fatty acids EPA and DHA are the second major category of nutrients that effectively complement Sirtfoods. Omega-3s have been the coveted natural wellbeing global favorite for years. What we didn't know before, which we are doing now, is that they also improve the activation of a group of sirtuin genes in the body that is directly linked to longevity. It makes them the perfect match for Sirtfoods.

Omega-3s have potent effects in decreasing inflammation and lowering fat blood levels. To that, we can add additional heart-healthy effects: rendering the blood less likely to pool, stabilizing the heart's electrical activity, and lowering blood pressure. Even the pharmaceutical industry now looks to them as an aid in the war against cardiac disease. And that is not where the litany of benefits ends. Omega-3s also have an effect on the way we perceive, having been shown to boost the outlook and help stave off dementia.

When we speak about omega-3s, we're thinking primarily about eating fish, particularly oily types, because no other dietary source comes close to supplying the significant levels of EPA and DHA that we need. And to see the benefits, all we need is two servings of fish a week, with an emphasis on oily fish. Sadly, the United States is not a country of big fish eaters, and that is accomplished by less than one in five Americans. As a result, our intake of the precious EPA and DHA is appallingly short.

Plant foods, including almonds, beans, and green leafy vegetables, often produce omega-3 but in a form called alpha-linolenic acid, which must be processed into EPA or DHA in the body. This conversion process is poor, meaning that alpha-linolenic acid delivers a negligible amount of our needs for omega-3. Even with the wonderful advantages of Sirtfoods, we shouldn't forget the added value that drinking adequate omega-3 fats provides. In that order, the best sources of omega-3 fish are herring, sardines, salmon, trout, and mackerel. While fresh tuna is naturally high, too, the tinned version loses the majority of the omega-3. And a replacement of DHA-enriched microalgae (up to 300 milligrams a day) is also recommended for vegetarians and vegans, though food foods should still be integrated into the diet.

10.5 Can A SirtFood Provide it All?

Our focus so far has been solely on Sirtfoods and reaping their maximum benefits in order to achieve the body we want and powerfully boost our health in the process. But is this a reasonable, long-term dietary solution to be taken? After all, there is more to diet than pure nutrients that trigger sirtuin. What about all the vitamins, minerals, and fibers that are also important to our wellbeing, and the diets that we should consume to satisfy such demands?

Based on sirtfood diets, augmented by protein-rich foods and omega-3 outlets, fulfill dietary needs across the entire spectrum of essential nutrients— much more so than any other diet does. They use kale, for example, because it is a good sirtfood, but it is a great source of vitamins C, folate, and manganese, calcium, Vitamin K and magnesium minerals. Kale is also a tremendous source of carotenoids lutein and zeaxanthin, both of which are critical for eye health, as well as immune-boosting beta-carotene.

Walnuts are also rich in minerals such as magnesium, copper, zinc, manganese, calcium, and iron, as well as fiber. Buckwheat is made of manganese, magnesium, zinc, potassium, and cotton. Tick the boxes of the onions for vitamin B6, folate, potassium, and food. Yet bananas, as well as potassium yet manganese, are good sources of vitamin C. And so, it begins. When you broaden your menu to include the expanded Sirtfood list and leave space for all the other good foods you enjoy eating, unwittingly, what you're going to end up with is a diet that's far richer in vitamins, nutrients, and fiber than you've ever had before. What Sirtfoods offers is a missing food group that changes the landscape of how we judge how good foods are for us, and how we eat a genuinely full diet.

10.6 The Physical Activity Effect

The Sirtfood Diet is about consuming certain products that are designed to promote sustainable weight loss and wellbeing by definition. But with the advantages that you see by practicing the plan, you can fall into the trap of feeling there's no need to exercise. This will be endorsed by many diet books, saying how ineffective exercise is compared with following the right diet for weight loss. And it's real; we can't outdo a bad diet. It's not the approach we saw earlier that was supposed to support weight loss. It's inefficient, and the harmfulness of being too many borders. So, it's that till we see stars or achieve an Olympian's feats, there's no need to pound the treadmill — but what about general everyday movement?

The truth is we are now much less involved than we used to be. The age of technology has ensured physical activity is practically factored out of our daily lives, for all the advancements it has provided. We don't have to mess with the whole process of being involved unless we want to. We can roll out of bed, drive to work, take the elevator, sit at a desk the whole day, drive home, eat and watch TV before rolling back into bed, then do the same the next day and the next day.

Forget about weight loss for a second and just glance at the litany of positive health benefits correlated with it. These include reduced risk of cardiovascular disease, stroke, hypertension, type 2 diabetes, osteoporosis, obesity and cancer, and improved mood, sleep, confidence, and a sense of wellbeing.

While many of the benefits of being active are driven by switching on our sirtuin genes, eating Sirtfoods shouldn't be used as a reason to not engage in exercise. Instead, we should understand how active the ideal complement to our Sirtfood intake is. It activates optimum stimulation of the sirtuin, and all the advantages that it provides, just as expected by definition.

What we are talking about here is meeting 150-minute (2 hours and 30 minutes) government guidelines of moderate physical activity a week. A moderate job is the equivalent of a brisk walk. But that doesn't have to be limited to this. Any sport or physical activity you love is fitting. Pleasure and exercise do not have to be mutually exclusive! So, their social aspect enriches squad or group sports even more. It's also about everyday things like taking the bike instead of the car, or getting off the bus one stop earlier, or just parking farther away to increase the distance you've got to walk around. Take the stairs and not the lift. Go outdoors and do gardening. Play in the park with your kids or get more out with the dog. Everything counts. Everything that has you up and moving will activate your sirtuin genes regularly and at moderate intensity, enhancing the benefits of the Sirtfood Diet.

Engaging in physical activity and eating a diet high in Sirtfood brings the buck the full sirtuin click. All it takes to achieve the benefit of physical activity is the equivalent of a quick 30-minute stroll five days a week.

SUMMARY

- Although the top twenty Sirtfoods should remain at the center of the plate, there are many other plants with sirtuin-activating properties that should be included in our diets to make them diverse and varied.

- A diet rich in Sirtfoods augmented by the addition of animal products and seafood offers all the advantages of triggering sirtuin, as well as satisfying the need for other essential nutrients.

- Although vegans and vegetarians can get all the benefits from a diet based on Sirtfood, careful attention should be paid to those nutrients that may be deficient, and correct food choices or supplements should be created.

Questions & Answers

1. If I am not fat, can I still follow this diet?

For anyone who is underweight, we do not prescribe Step 1 of the Sirtfood Diet. A simple way to find out that if you are underweight is to measure the body mass index. As long as you are aware of your height and weight, you can quickly determine using any number of online BMI calculators. If your BMI is 18 or less, we do not recommend embarking on the diet phase 1. They would still urge caution if your BMI is between 18.5 and 20, as adopting the diet can imply that your BMI drop below 18.5. While many people aspire to be super-skinny, the reality is that underweight can have a negative impact on many health aspects, contributing to a lower immune system, an increased risk of osteoporosis (weakening bones), and fertility issues. While phase 1 of the diet is not recommended if you are underweight, we still encourage the integration of plenty of Sirtfoods into a balanced way of eating so that all the health benefits of these foods can be reaped. If you're slim but have a healthy range of BMI (20–25), however, there's absolutely nothing to stop you from getting started. A majority of the pilot trial participants had BMI in the healthy range, but still lost impressive amounts of weight and got more toned. Importantly, many of them reported significantly improved levels and appearance of the energy. Sirtfood diet is about promoting health just as much as weight-loss.

2. If you take any medications, so is it fine to follow this diet?

The Sirtfood Diet is suitable for most people. Still, due to its powerful effects on fat burning and health, it can alter the processes of certain diseases and the medication actions prescribed by your doctor. Similarly, certain medicines are not suitable in a state of fasting. During the Sirtfood Diet trial, we assessed each individual's suitability before they embarked on the diet, particularly those taking medication. We can't do that for you, so if you have a significant health problem, are taking prescribed medicines or have other reasons to worry about getting on a diet, we recommend that you discuss it with your doctor.

3. If someone's expecting, still can follow this diet?

If you are trying to conceive or are pregnant or breastfeeding, we do not recommend embarking on the Sirtfood Diet. It is a powerful diet for weight loss which makes it inappropriate. Don't be put off eating plenty of Sirtfoods, though, as these are exceptionally healthy foods to be included as part of a balanced and varied pregnancy diet. Because of its alcohol content, you will want to avoid red wine and limit caffeinated items such as coffee, green tea, and cocoa not to exceed 200 milligrams of caffeine per day during pregnancy (one mug of instant coffee typically contains about 100 milligrams of caffeine). Recommendations should not surpass four cups of green tea per day and should skip matcha altogether. Other than that, you can reap the benefits of incorporating sirt foods into your diet.

4. How often can I repeat Phase 1 and Phase 2?

Phase 1 can be repeated if you feel a weight loss or health boost is needed. To ensure long-term adverse effects of calorie restriction on your metabolism are not present, you should wait at least a month before repeating. But in fact, we find that most people at most need to repeat in no more frequently than once in every three months and continue to get incredible results. Instead, if you find that you've gone off-track, need some fine-tuning, or want a bit more sirtfood intensity, we recommend repeating as often as you like some or all days of the Phase 2 section. Phase 2 is, after all, about establishing a lifelong way to eat. Remember, the Sirtfood Diet's beauty is that it doesn't require you to feel like you're endlessly on a diet. Still, instead, it's the springboard to developing positive lifelong dietary changes that create a lighter, leaner, healthier you.

5. I have heard many times about superfoods, should I include these in my diet?

The first thing you need to know about the term superfood is that it's a marketing slogan and not a scientific term at all. You don't need to think about so-called superfoods because the Sirtfood Diet puts together the planet's healthiest foods into a revolutionary new way of eating. Just as relying on a simple vitamin pill to make us healthy is a mistake, so building on a single superfood to do the same is also a mistake. It is the entire diet, consisting of a broad spectrum of Sirtfoods and their vast array of natural compounds, acting in synergy, which is the real secret to achieving weight loss and lifelong health.

6. Should I exercise during Phase 1?

Regular exercising is the best things you can do for your health and doing some moderate exercise will enhance the diet's phase 1 weight-loss and health benefits. In general, we advise you to maintain your usual level of exercise and physical activity through the Sirtfood Diet's first seven days. However, we suggest staying in your normal comfort zone, as prolonged or excessively intense exercise can simply put too much stress on the body during this period. Eye your body. There's no need to push yourself during Phase 1 for more exercise; instead, let the Sirtfoods do the hard work.

7. I am fat, is sirtfood diet best for me?

Yeah! Don't be upset by the fact that only a small minority of our pilot study participants were obese. This is because the pilot study was conducted in a health and fitness club where people are usually fitter and more aware of their well-being. Instead, be encouraged by the fact that the few who were obese had even better results than our healthy-weight participants. There are a lot of people of people who tried the diet in the real world replicated those results. You should also stand to reap the most significant changes in your well-being, based on the research into sirtuin activation. Getting obese increases the risk of many chronic health problems, and these are the very diseases against which Sirtfoods helps to protect.

8. If I get the best results and reached my target weight, so should I stop eating sirtfoods?

Firstly, many congratulations on your success in terms of weight loss! With Sirtfoods, you've had great success, but it doesn't end now. While we do not advocate more restrictions on calories, your diet should still have enough Sirtfood. Many of our consumers are now at their ideal body shape continue to eat diets high in Sirtfood. The great thing about Sirtfoods is they are a lifestyle. In terms of weight management, the best way to think about them is that they help bring the body to the weight and composition it was intended to be. They work from here to preserve and hold you are looking great and feeling great. Essentially, this is the aim we wish for all adherents of the Sirtfood Diet.

9. I have finished phase 2, so now should I stop drinking sirtfood green juice in the morning?

The green juice is our favorite way to start the day with a fantastic hit from Sirtfoods, so we endorse its long-term consumption. Our Sirtfood green juice has been carefully designed to include ingredients that provide a full spectrum of sirtuin-activating nutrients in potent dose-boosting fat-burning and wellness. We're all for variety, however, and while we recommend that you continue with a morning juice, we fully support anyone looking to experiment with various Sirtfood juice concoctions.

10. Are sirtfoods suitable for children?

The Sirtfood Diet is a powerful diet for weight loss and not intended for kids. That doesn't mean that kids should miss out on the excellent health benefits offered by including more Sirtfoods in their overall diet, though. For babies, a vast majority of Sirtfoods reflect incredibly healthy foods and help them achieve good and nutritious diets. Many of the meals planned for the diet's Phase 2 have been developed with families in mind, including the taste buds of babies. The likes of the Sirtfood pizza, the chili con carne, and the Sirtfood bites are perfect child-friendly foods with a nutritional value higher than usual children's food offerings. While most Sirtfoods are incredibly healthy for children to eat, the green juice that is too rich in fat-burning sirtfoods is not approved. We also advise against important caffeine sources, such as coffee and green tea. You will also need to be vigilant of chilies being included and may choose to keep things milder for kids.

11. Will I get any headache or feel tired during phase 1?

Phase 1 of the Sirtfood Diet offers strong naturally occurring food compounds in quantities that most people wouldn't get through their healthy diet, and some people will respond when they adjust to this drastic dietary shift. This may include symptoms such as mild headache or tiredness, although these effects are minor and short-lived in our experience. Of course, if the signs are serious or give you cause for concern, we suggest that you seek medical advice promptly. We have never seen anything other than occasional mild symptoms that quickly resolve, and within a few days, most people find that they have a renewed sense of energy, vigor, and well-being.

12. Should I take any supplements?

Unless your doctor or another health-care professional prescribe explicitly for you, we do not recommend indiscriminate use of nutritional supplements. You will be ingesting from Sirtfoods a vast and synergistic array of natural plant compounds, and it is these that will do you good. You cannot duplicate such benefits with nutritional supplements, and some nutritional supplements, such as antioxidants, can potentially conflict with the beneficial effects of Sirtfoods, which is the last thing you want, particularly if taken at high doses. Whenever possible, we think that getting the nutrients you need from eating a balanced diet rich in Sirtfoods is much better than taking the nutrients in the form of a pill. However, Vegans will have special nutritional considerations and our specific recommendations for those following diets which are purely plant-based. Furthermore, since plant proteins are lower in leucine, the amino acid that enhances Sirtfoods' actions, we have found that vegans can benefit from supplementing their diet with appropriate vegan protein powder. It refers in turn to those who perform high levels of exercise. This supplement should be taken off the Sirtfood green juice at a separate time of day.

13. Does the Sirtfood diet provide enough amount of fibers?

Many Sirtfoods are, of course, rich fibers. Onions, endive, and walnuts are popular examples, with buckwheat and Medjool dates mainly sticking out, suggesting the fiber department is not deprived of a Sirtfood-rich diet. Even in Phase 1, when food consumption is reduced, most of us will still consume the amount of fiber we're used to, especially if we select from the menu options the recipes that contain buckwheat, beans, and lentils. Nonetheless, for others reported to be vulnerable to intestinal problems such as constipation without higher intakes of fiber, an appropriate fiber supplement may be recommended during Phase 1, particularly Days 1 to 3, which should be addressed with your health care professional.

14. Is it mandatory to do phase 1 for seven days – can I do fewer?

There is nothing magical about seven days in Phase 1. Simply that is what we decided for our trial. We went for that because it was long enough to produce impressive results, but not long enough to make things arduous. It fits neatly into the lives of people as well. It was tested for seven days and what is proven to be effective. However, if you want to cut it short by a day or two for whatever reason, do so by completing until the end of Day 5 or Day 6. Don't worry, the lion's share of the benefits will still be reaped.

References

- Haigis, M. C., & Guarente, L. P. (2006). Mammalian sirtuins—emerging roles in physiology, aging, and calorie restriction. *Genes & development, 20*(21), 2913-2921.
- Aragonès, G., Ardid-Ruiz, A., Ibars, M., Suárez, M., & Bladé, C. (2016). Modulation of leptin resistance by food compounds. *Molecular nutrition & food research, 60*(8), 1789-1803.
- Ryall, J. G., Dell'Orso, S., Derfoul, A., Juan, A., Zare, H., Feng, X., ... & Sartorelli, V. (2015). The NAD+-dependent SIRT deacetylase translates a metabolic switch into regulatory epigenetics in skeletal muscle stem cells. *Cell stem cell, 16*(2), 171-183.
- Wilking, M. J., & Ahmad, N. (2015). The role of SIRT in cancer: the saga continues. *The American journal of pathology, 185*(1), 26.
- Si, H., & Liu, D. (2014). Dietary antiaging phytochemicals and mechanisms associated with prolonged survival. *The Journal of nutritional biochemistry, 25*(6), 581-591.
- Duarte, D. A., Mariana Ap B, R., Papadimitriou, A., Silva, K. C., Amancio, V. H. O., Mendonça, J. N., ... & de Faria, J. M. L. (2015). Polyphenol-enriched cocoa protects the diabetic retina from glial reaction through the sirtuin pathway. *The Journal of nutritional biochemistry, 26*(1), 64-74.
- Luccarini, I., Pantano, D., Nardiello, P., Cavone, L., Lapucci, A., Miceli, C., ... & Casamenti, F. (2016). The polyphenol oleuropein aglycone modulates the PARP1-SIRT interplay: an in vitro and in vivo study. *Journal of Alzheimer's Disease, 54*(2), 737-750.
- Ibarrola-Jurado, N., Bulló, M., Guasch-Ferré, M., Ros, E., Martínez-González, M. A., Corella, D., ... & Arós, F. (2013).

Cross-sectional assessment of nut consumption and obesity, metabolic syndrome and other cardiometabolic risk factors: the PREDIMED study. *PloS one, 8*(2).

- Yao, K., Duan, Y., Li, F., Tan, B., Hou, Y., Wu, G., & Yin, Y. (2016). Leucine in obesity: therapeutic prospects. *Trends in pharmacological sciences, 37*(8), 714-727.
- Hosseini, A., & Hosseinzadeh, H. (2015). A review on the effects of Allium sativum (Garlic) in metabolic syndrome. *Journal of endocrinological investigation, 38*(11), 1147-1157.
- Baliga, M. S., Baliga, B. R. V., Kandathil, S. M., Bhat, H. P., & Vayalil, P. K. (2011). A review of the chemistry and pharmacology of the date fruits (Phoenix dactylifera L.). *Food research international, 44*(7), 1812-1822.
- Niseteo, T., Komes, D., Belščak-Cvitanović, A., Horžić, D., & Budeč, M. (2012). Bioactive composition and antioxidant potential of different commonly consumed coffee brews affected by their preparation technique and milk addition. *Food chemistry, 134*(4), 1870-1877.
- Aune, D., Navarro Rosenblatt, D. A., Chan, D. S., Vieira, A. R., Vieira, R., Greenwood, D. C., ... & Norat, T. (2015). Dairy products, calcium, and prostate cancer risk: a systematic review and meta-analysis of cohort studies. *The American journal of clinical nutrition, 101*(1), 87-117.
- Melnik, B. C. (2015). Milk—a nutrient system of mammalian evolution promoting mTORC1-dependent translation. *International journal of molecular sciences, 16*(8), 17048-17087.

information contained within this book, either directly or indirectly.

Legal Notice:

This book is copyright protected. It is only for personal use. You cannot amend, distribute, sell, use, quote or paraphrase any part, or the content within this book, without the consent of the author or publisher.

Disclaimer Notice:

Please note the information contained within this document is for educational and entertainment purposes only. All effort has been executed to present accurate, up to date, reliable, complete information. No warranties of any kind are declared or implied. Readers acknowledge that the author is not engaging in the rendering of legal, financial, medical or professional advice. The content within this book has been derived from various sources. Please consult a licensed professional before attempting any techniques outlined in this book.

By reading this document, the reader agrees that under no circumstances is the author responsible for any losses, direct or indirect, that are incurred as a result of the use of information contained within this document, including, but not limited to, errors, omissions, or inaccuracies.

Introduction

Fasting has been around for millennia. It has played important roles in religious and medical literature for nearly as long. In many modern religions, fasting is the way to create spiritual connection, to find guidance or to improve mindfulness. Fasts that automatically come to mind are Lent in Catholisim and Orthodox Christianity, Ramadan in Islam or meditation fasts is some Buddhist schools. Lent lasts 40 days, and while some churches may allow more freedom with the fast, traditionally Lent required a fast where only one meal a day was eaten. During Ramadan, a month long fast, Muslims don't eat while the sun is up and then eat once the sun is down. Essentially, it is an eight to 12 hour fast, with some time to eat at night and early in the morning. In some Buddhist schools, fasting takes place to aid in meditation and spiritual practices. This often happens everyday, with the dinner meal skipped. So within religions and spiritual practices, there are many different kinds of fasts.

People have also fasted for political reasons. Perhaps

most famously is Gandhi and his social protests. He fasted multiple times to protest a variety of social issues in India. There have been other hunger-strikes throughout history, where people fasted to create political change including suffragette fasting in Europe and the U.S. Many political fasts promote a feeling of guilt in those watching, and can result in change, though it has often resulted in death as well.

Medically, fasting has been around since the time of Hippocrates. Fasting was prescribed during times when the patient was sick enough that eating was considered detrimental. Past physicians believed that fasting would help with the healing of injuries and diseases. While it's unclear whether this was actually true, today, modern fasting is associated with better health improvements. In fact, intermittent fasting is our modern take on fasting for healing.

Intermittent fasting is when you choose not to eat for a specific amount of time. For example, you might fast during the evening and night hours, or you might fast every other day. In general, intermittent fasting doesn't go beyond a day of fasting. So you won't see many intermittent fasts that are 30 hours of fasting or longer. Despite how it may sound, intermittent fasting is not starvation and in fact, it's quite healthy. Intermittent fasts are about improving your health. In general, it can benefit people who are looking to lose weight, improve their blood sugar levels, and reduce their insulin resistance.

In this book, we'll cover the basics of intermittent fasting. We'll explore the different kinds, from the everyday ease of the 14/10 method to the difficult but rewarding alternate-day fast. We'll also discuss who is a perfect candidate for trying intermittent fasting, and who should refrain from it. We'll go over the benefits and risks, and explore associated research studies that demonstrate the effectiveness of intermittent fasting. Finally, we'll go into detail about schedules and possible menus for starting intermittent fasting. With this book, you'll get a thorough introduction to intermittent fasting and you'll begin your journey to starting your own intermittent fast. Let's begin.

Chapter 1: Basics of Intermittent Fasting

The beauty of social media is that ideas can be shared around the world and gain popularity very quickly. It's probably why you're here, reading this book. On social media you can find many influencers and celebrities who have tried intermittent fasting, and wholeheartedly advocate for it. Whether you want to look like the actors who play superheroes or whether you just want to get healthier, intermittent fasting can help you achieve your goals.

In the introduction, we covered how fasting was used throughout history for health, political, religious reasons. Some of these fasts are very similar to intermittent fasting. In general, intermittent fasting is when you time your eating to fit within a specific window during your day or week. Your fasting hours might just be during the night, or they might extend to a full 24 hours. When comparing intermittent fasting to religious fasting, you will see some similarities with Ramadan and Lent. During Ramadan, most people don't eat during the day, and instead eat all their meals at night. This is very similar to a 16/8 fast or even a 20/4 fast, where eating takes place in a small eight or four hour window at night. Depending on the style of Lent a person follows, you may only have one large meal in the day instead of many meals. Or you may only eat for some portion of the week and fast completely on other days. This can also be quite like intermittent fasting schedules. The difference between religious fasts and intermittent fasting are, of course, the purpose but also the timing. Religious fasts often take place for a short period of time like 20-40 days, but intermittent fasting can be a whole lifestyle change, and result in you fasting for years! It's not necessary to do it for the long term, but many people continue it even when they meet their goals for fasting.

There are so many different varieties of intermittent fasting that you'll have and easy way of finding one that fits into your lifestyle. In general, there are the methods that require you to eat in a small window everyday. These are the methods like the 12/12, 14/10, 16/8, and 20/4. In these methods, the first number is how many hours you fast, and the second number is how many hours are in your eating window. You would eat all your meals during that window of time, and during the fasting point, you would just drink liquids. The other types of fasts are those that include 24 hours of fasting between eating days. Some of these do calorie restricted meals during the fasting period so that hunger doesn't become overwhelming. Methods that do the longer 24 hour fast (with or without small meals on fasting days) include alternate day fasts, the 5:2 fast, and a general 24 hour fast. Alternate day fasts and 5:2 fasts can be similar as they take place during the course of one week. However, alternate day fasts require fasting three or four days of the week, alternating your eating days and your fasting days. While the 5:2 fast is eating normally for five days with two days of fasting spread out within the week. The 24 hour fast is one you might do once a week or even just once a month! Whichever fast you choose to do, you'll want to choose one that fits your daily life. We'll discuss these kinds of fasts later in the book.

It's important to mention that intermittent fasting isn't a diet. While people use it to receive health benefits (like they do for dieting), intermittent fasting isn't a diet at all. Most diets are focused on *what* you eat, however, intermittent fasting is all about *when* you eat. It focuses on the timing of eating to change your body's current state and bring it more into homeostasis. This can sound a little fantasy-like. Afterall, how can changing the times you eat help? Well, there's a lot of research out there about intermittent fasting, and depending on the type of fasting you follow, intermittent fasting can change your metabolism, insulin levels, and more. Let's explore more about why intermittent fasting works.

Why it Works

I can tell you that you'll lose weight on intermittent fasting and you'll become healthier. But none of that explains why? Why does fasting have such positive reviews and a following? Intermittent fasting works for so many reasons, but the main ones are the fact that it can fit in your daily life, changes some of your physiology, and can result in some caloric restriction.

Fits your life

Diets can cause a lot of changes your life. They often require specific foods that must be eaten. This can be frustrating if you live in an area where some foods aren't available. It can also be frustrating cost wise, as a lot of diet foods can be quite expensive. All of these can impact your motivation to continue dieting. Intermittent fasting doesn't cause this change to your life. You don't have to eat specific types of food when fasting. Nor do you have to spend a fortune following the schedule. All it requires of you is to eat at a specific time of day, and eat healthy meals during your eating window. This can ease the strain of starting a new fasting schedule. This also means that you won't have to do a huge change to your lifestyle.

Cravings can be a nightmare when following other styles of dieting. You can follow a low calorie diet, but you'll probably miss eating that burger from your favorite shop, or having a scoop of ice cream with your kids. You could follow a very low or no carb diet, but you might end up missing bread, and feel a lot of restrictions when it comes to choosing your food. This can reduce the sustainability of dieting in your life. Intermittent fasting can be more reliable because you're not going to have any cravings. It doesn't restrict what you eat, which is honestly the hardest part of most conventional diets. By not restricting what you eat, you're not likely to struggle with cravings. Depending on which fasting method you choose, you might struggle with hunger, but probably not cravings.

Many of us don't follow a set eating schedule. We will often find ourselves skipping meals when we get into the flow of work or when we oversleep. Because we don't have set times to eat normally, it's really easy to change our schedule at the drop of a hat. That's why some intermittent fasts can fit into your daily schedule. If you only have to shift your eating a bit during the day, you will not struggle with the change so much. For example, if you choose to follow the 14/10 fasting schedule, you'll only have to shift your breakfast and dinner times by a couple of hours. That's so easy! Other methods of fasting can be easier, or harder depending on your current lifestyle.

Intermittent fasting doesn't require a huge shift in how

you eat, unlike some other diets, which is why it can be easier to follow and fit your lifestyle better than conventional (or unconventional) diets.

Caloric restriction

Another reason that fasting works is because it can result in some unplanned calorie restriction. Calorie restriction is one of the reasons people lose weight in a regular low calorie diet. Unplanned calorie restriction means that you have a slightly lower number of daily or weekly calories than you normally eat during the day or week. Normally, an adult who is of average height and weight, eats between 2000-2200 calories a day. When fasting, you might have difficulty eating as much as you normally do during the day. Afterall, you only have a small eating window in some fasting methods. So you may end up eating 1800 calories a day. This is a significant reduction in calories, and it's all unplanned. By having this reduction, you're guaranteed to lose some weight while fasting.

In some methods of fasting, you might have some planned caloric restriction. The 24 hour methods which result in 24 hours without food, obviously result in significant weekly calorie reductions. If a healthy adult of average height and weight eats 14,000 - 15,400 calories per week, then by having some 24 hour fasts can reduce that by 2,000-6,000 calories, depending on the type of fast you choose. Alternate day fasting will provide you with way more calorie reductions than other fasts. Again, all of this reduction will result in weight loss. Because some fasts can be easier than following a consistent calorie reduction diet, fasting for this purpose can give you some good results without causing a lot of pain.

Changes your physiology

This one is a little complicated and will be discussed extensively in the chapter on benefits and risks. However, to give you a basic overview, intermittent fasting works because it can change some of your physiology and put your body back to homeostasis. By shifting your eating times, you force your body to change the way it uses its stores of glucose. This results in your body shifting from burning glucose as fuel to burning fat because the glucose stores have been used up during the fasting window. This leads to a whole host of health benefits. The best part is that these health benefits continue even after you're back to eating during your eating window. Fasting can also change your hormone levels, which also help your health and can provide so many benefits, especially to those who are already struggling with health issues. We'll cover all of this more in the chapter on benefits and risks.

Fasting is for…Everyone?

Intermittent fasting can sound rather fantastic and easy. But don't let its simple description fool you. It's a process and it can be difficult to stick with. Because of this, it's important to consider fasting carefully before you try it. Despite how much I wish I could say that fasting is for everyone, this simply isn't true. Fasting works for some, and for others it can be a dangerous affair. Here are some people who should and who should not try intermittent fasting. As always, please follow your doctor's recommendation about intermittent fasting before starting.

Let's say you already live a pretty healthy life. You exercise regularly, eat healthy meals, and are generally untroubled by any illnesses, mental or physical. If this describes you, then you could go ahead and try your fasting method of choice. You probably wouldn't have many or any side effects because you already know the basics of doing the best for your body. However, if you're like the rest of us, who have lived off fast food for most of our lives and are looking for a change, you should consider your general health and discipline towards a fast before starting. Whatever your current health status is, there are some things you should consider before starting a fast.

Consider your social priorities before you start fasting. Many people enjoy meals with their friends and family on the weekends. We also tend to eat meals with our children in the evenings. So, once you've chosen a method you're interested in, you'll need to consider how you are going to schedule your meals to fit your social engagements. If you're doing a daily fast with a method like 14/10 or 20/4, think about when you'll end your fast. Also consider if your family will be following your pattern, or if you'll be going it alone. If you're the one cooking for your family, will you be able to handle any cravings that come from watching them eat while you don't? Essentially, just consider the impact on your day to day eating habits. This will help you narrow down types of fasting that will work for you.

Beyond the social considerations, you'll have to consider your support system. It's really empowering to have people cheering for you when you're doing something hard, or new. Think about going to college and having a support system. It's so much easier than going alone. Fasting can be very difficult, and while you can go it alone, it's easier with a support system in place. This is especially true if you're planning on this being a lifestyle change. So, go through your phone contacts, and pick a few people who are reliable and can offer you support and encouragement while you start your fast. These are the people who won't make you feel guilty about not eating when they eat. They're the people who will encourage you when all you want to do is eat cake at midnight during your fasting hours. They're the people who may even choose to fast with you! Just have a support system. Furthermore, if you don't have a support system in your daily life, create your own support system by becoming active in online support groups and health coaching groups.

This is a more practical consideration but think about how your emotions might change as you fast. The first change in your eating schedule can lead to some changed moods. You might even have a change in your sleeping habits. These changes, though different, are related and can affect your life. You might be tired at work and being tired makes you feel very hungry. You may have feelings of anger when you're hungry (commonly known as being 'hangry'). You may have other shifts in your mood, but it's different for everyone. You'll need to make plans for adapting to your body's changes before starting your fast. This will help your adjustment period.

One final consideration is for anyone who does a lot of exercise or workouts. You can exercise while on your fast, but you'll need to be slow and careful when transitioning into your fast. You'll probably have to change how much protein and fiber you eat. You'll also need to plan your exercising window to coincide with your eating window. You don't want to exercise and then fast for 10 hours. Instead, you want to make sure that you have a meal after you exercise so that your body can recover. If you're an athlete, you're going to want to talk with your doctor to see if intermittent fasting will be beneficial for you before starting.

While it's important to take all of these things into consideration, fasting still isn't helpful for everyone. Here are people who shouldn't be fasting:

- Those who are pregnant or want to be pregnant.

- Those who have experienced eating disorders, anxiety, or depression (not without a doctor's recommendation).

- Those who have some medical illnesses (again, not without a doctor's recommendation).

- Those who are children. Seriously. Anyone under the age of 18 probably shouldn't fast.

Let's look at these demographics in detail to explain why

fasting won't work for people in them.

Pregnancy is possibly one of the only times in your life when you can eat whatever you want, and people won't stop you. That might not be healthy though, so it's easy to see how you may want to lose weight while pregnant. But fasting is not the way to go. Being pregnant means that you are providing the necessary nutrition for both you and your baby. Your baby's development depends entirely on what you put in your body. Fasting will result in you not intaking the right amount of food for both of you. This can negatively affect your child's development. Just like how drinking alcohol or smoking while pregnant can result in detrimental fetal development, so too can fasting. If your heart is set on trying intermittent fasting, then please try it after your baby has been weaned and you're both healthy.

If you're trying to get pregnant, then don't do intermittent fasting. There has been a couple animal studies with intermittent fasting that resulted in females having changed menstruation, low fertility, and skipped periods. While this research hasn't been carried over to humans, you don't really want to take the risk. So, wait to start intermittent fasting until another time in your life.

Intermittent fasting can mess around with your hormones. It will shift your mood at the beginning. This can be dangerous for those who already struggle with mental illnesses or past mental illnesses. Fasting can push you into a relapse of anxiety or depression because of the change in your hormone levels. If you've experienced anxiety or depression before, you should talk to your doctor before trying fasting. You should also set up checks with your support system so they can identify if you're becoming more anxious or depressed while on a fast.

If you have ever had an eating disorder, you shouldn't fast at all. Eating disorders are all about having a really bad relationship with food, and even if you've recovered, fasting can push you back into disordered eating. Anorexia, bulimia, and binge eating are all different kinds of disordered eating. Doing a fast while experiencing one of these disorders, or after recovering from one, can push you back into disordered eating. It's easy to start fasting and then just keep going without enough eating windows if you've already experienced anorexia. Fasting could also cause a flare in binge eating when breaking your fast because you're hungry from not eating for several hours. Both these situations are dangerous for your body and your mental state. So if you have experienced an eating disorder, fasting is not recommended at all, not even with a doctor's recommendation. Please don't endanger your mental health just to try and improve your physical health.

Intermittent fasting can have some good benefits for your body. If you are already struggling with some medical issues, you need to take a moment to step back and reassess your fasting ideas. Fasting can help with insulin resistance, so if you're pre-diabetic or even have been recently diagnosed with type 2 diabetes, intermittent fasting can help you, though your doctor should discuss it with you first. However, if you have been diagnosed with diabetes for a while, and have already experienced significant damage from it, then intermittent fasting shouldn't be pursued. The reason being that fasting changes your metabolic rate, insulin levels, and blood-sugar levels. If you're already struggling with maintaining these things, then fasting will throw you for a loop. Talk to your doctor if you're concerned about your weight, and they can give you some good advice for approaching a diet change or fast. Please don't just jump right in.

While diabetes is the primary concern when approaching fasting, if you have any medical difficulties, you should really talk to your doctor.

The final demographic of people who should not fast are children. There are a lot of reasons why children shouldn't fast. One of them is about people and their relationship to food. As children, we learn about food, how it makes us feel, and grow attachments to our eating habits. These habits can follow us into adulthood. Just think about it: What food brings you comfort? What do you eat when you're sad or angry? When did you learn that? A lot of this comes from childhood and what we learned during it. Comfort food literally comforts us, and the food item can be different for each person. So what we learn about food as children can follow us. If what children learn is to restrict eating, then they're not going to learn about good relationships with food. As they grow older, it will always be about restricting food. This can lead to another problem.

If children fast while growing, they'll learn that food should be restricted. This can create disordered eating, specifically anorexia. We've already discussed the importance of not fasting if you've experienced anorexia. But it's critical that children aren't taught restrictive eating in case they end up not eating at all. Now of course, fasting will not automatically cause anorexia. But it can be a trigger. Children have disordered eating for a lot of reasons, but it all narrows down to have an 'ideal' body type. If children think that fasting can get them there, then they may choose to go beyond fasting and into starvation. So it's critically important that children don't fast.

To wrap up this chapter, I urge you to first talk to your doctor before fasting. This recommendation is for anyone who is unsure about how fasting will help them, or anyone who has a current health condition. Your doctor will be able to tell you definitively about whether fasting is for you or not and help ensure that you won't affect your health negatively during your fast. Fasting can benefit a lot of people, but it's not for everyone. In the next few chapters, we're going to explore more about fasting. First, we will tackle those pesky myths you've probably heard about fasting. After that, we will examine the benefits and risks of fasting, as well as the studies that support its effectiveness. Before choosing whether you want to fast or not, check out these next two chapters. They provide some awesome information that may persuade you to try fasting.

Chapter 2: Myths of Intermittent Fasting

Myths are a beautiful thing. They're presented as absolute fact, without any proof, and we're all expected to believe them. However, they often don't have any sort of basis and can easily be debunked with just a little knowledge. This strange nature of myth can create some of our greatest stories. But in our more modern era, myths can change our beliefs and influence our decisions. Think about a lot of the myths, and often straight up lies, sent out over social media and how they negatively affect people. Myths like these can change the way we do business, take care of our families, or even approach politics or religion. The most amazing thing about myths is that we all believe them. It doesn't matter how much of a skeptic you are, there is at least one myth that you believe in. As our society keeps creating more myths, there are more and more opportunities for you to believe things that are simply untrue. This chapter is all about making sure you don't believe the myths associated with intermittent fasting.

Anytime that you have a new experience or a new idea,

there are always going to be people who are willing to poke holes in it or make things up about it. I could say, "Intermittent fasting is a cure all for everything! Have appendicitis? Fast! Have a headache? Fast! Getting a little heavy while pregnant? Fast! It will solve all your problems!" And you could choose to believe me. But really, without proof you wouldn't know if I've just made these statements up or not (and yes, I did make them up, please don't fast if you're pregnant). If you choose to believe many of the other myths about fasting, then you can miss out on some great opportunities with fasting. Or worse, you could hurt yourself if you believe some of the myths. So it's important to fact check before following believing and follow myths.

While intermittent fasting is a bit new, there are still a lot of myths about it. Before starting with intermittent fasting, it's important to go through the myths so that you know exactly what is fact and what is fiction about intermittent fasting. Because we want you to believe us when we say that fasting can be beneficial, we'll include the sources for this information and research studies associated with each myth.

Myth #1: Fasting is the Same as Starvation

When many people think about fasting, they think about starvation. After all, if you're not eating, then you must be starving. However, this myth isn't true. We fast every day, for about eight hours as we sleep, and yet we don't starve. You can even skip a meal on top of your sleep time, and not starve. Beyond just this basic daily fast we all do, starvation changes our body in a different way in comparison to intermittent fasting.

In the U.S. starvation is uncommon, though it's more common to have some food insecurity. If you are experiencing starvation, you'll have not eaten for a while, or eaten very low calorie meals for several days. In fact, your starvation response starts after merely three days of not eating enough calories (Berg, Tymoczko, & Strye, 2002). During this time, you will lose weight, but you will also damage your body. In this case, your body and your brain know that you're starving, and they decide to try and save you. So your brain slows down your metabolism and sends out hormones to make you very hungry. Your body starts looking for food elsewhere. Now the science behind starvation is really detailed, but suffice it to say, normally our body gets its energy from our food, which increases our blood-glucose levels, and our insulin — all of which feeds our body. However, when starving, our body runs out of its stores of glucose and starts searching for other sources of energy. In the search for protein, your body will start cannibalizing itself, eating through important cells, and muscles. It's not a quick process, because your body still needs to function to find more food. However, without food, your body will slowly lose its functionality, leading to death.

Most of us won't starve to death in the U.S. Even when eating a very low calorie diet, our body will keep pushing us to eat and with a lot of access to food, even if most is unhealthy, we're not likely to starve to death. However, we can still feel the effects of the starvation response without the right nutrition during the day. Not only will our brain keep sending out hunger warnings, but we'll also have a shift in emotions and sometimes, cognitive function. Researchers during WWII studied starvation to determine how our bodies react to it. This study is known as the Minnesota Starvation Experiment (Keys et al., 1950), and it found some interesting effects on our brains from starvation. Many of the participants experienced emotional swings, felt cognitively foggy, and had dreams about food. They became depressed, anxious, and irritable. Physically, they experienced fluctuating body temperature, felt weak, and had reduced stamina. Their heart rate also decreased. These effects were felt in a stage of semi-starvation, where they were eating, but only a little everyday and very little of what they ate was healthy. So even when having food, we can experience the effects of starvation.

Intermittent fasting is very different from starvation because you won't be without food for three days. In fact, so long as you're following a set, healthy, fasting schedule, you will only be without food for 24 hours or less. So you will not to initiate your natural starvation response. Our body is used to normal fasting, eating states. Once you eat your last meal before a fast, your body has high blood-sugar levels, and increased insulin which are all fueling your body. The body also stores the extra glucose and puts it aside for later. After the first several hours, your body starts to reduce it's insulin levels and your blood-sugar levels also drop. Your liver releases it's stores of glucose and then your body starts using fatty tissue to continue fueling itself since it's blood-sugar levels are lower. This state is known as ketosis. Your body remains in this state for a while, even when you eat again (Berg, Tymoczko, & Strye, 2002). Because you're providing your body with food, even after 24 hours without, your body doesn't shift into its starvation response. Instead, it sticks with its stage of ketosis, with reduced insulin levels and blood-sugar levels, before getting more energy from your next meal.

It's important to note that while there are differences between starvation and fasting, any fast taken for too long will result in starvation. Any diet, where you are eating less than 1000 calories a day, puts you at risk for starting your body's starvation response. However, this response won't happen immediately. So long as you are eating something during your days, you'll be ok. In most fasts, you're going to eat your regular daily calories every day. But in some fasts like the 5:2 and the Alternate Day fasting, you'll have periods of low-calorie intake. Even during these periods, you'll only be without food for 24 hours or less. So, while doing intermittent fasting, your body shouldn't have a starvation response.

Myth #2: Fasting will Make You Gain Weight

This myth is closely related to the previous myth. It's connected to the starvation response, or as many people call it, "Starvation Mode." Starvation mode is the same thing as our starvation response, but just in a more sensationalized perspective. The general myth most people have is that fasting will put you into starvation mode, which means your metabolism slows down, you'll start hoarding all the fuel your body takes in because of the slow metabolism, and thus, you'll gain weight. Let's break this down because it's a complicated myth.

We've already covered how fasting won't put you into starvation mode if it's done correctly. So we're going to explore the metabolism aspect. When you're starving, and your body/brain starts trying to save itself, it starts to lower it's metabolism. Your metabolism is what helps you maintain your body's weight and repair your cells. It's how your body processes the food you eat and turns it into the fuel used to power your every action. During starvation, your metabolism rate will reduce because you don't have enough food to keep it running at its optimal level. This is to conserve energy for your most important living functions. Because people often think that fasting is the same as starvation, they expect your metabolism to slow while fasting, resulting in you gaining weight. This is confusing because during starvation, yes, your metabolic rate decreases, but your body is using all the stores it has. This means that there isn't any extra fuel! You will not gain weight when you're starving. It's impossible. So, carrying that belief over to fasting, just doesn't work.

In most diet culture, you'll hear people talk about 'fast' metabolism and 'slow' metabolism. Having a fast metabolism is supposed to help you lose weight because you're burning more food and fuel than you're eating and storing. A slow metabolism is supposed to make you gain weight because you're not burning enough fuel and everything extra you eat gets stored. So when people think about this myth, they think that your lack of food, will reduce your metabolism, which will lead to more food storage, with less energy and stores being used. However, this isn't true with fasting. Fasting improves your metabolism and uses your stores of energy efficiently (Patterson et al., 2016). Done right, it's likely that you will lose weight when fasting, not gain weight.

While I'd like to fully debunk this myth, there is some truth to it, and it all comes down to diet. It's possible that you can gain weight when fasting, but it's not because of your metabolic rate. If you choose to eat regular meals that exceed your daily calories, then you're going to gain weight. This is the same with any diet, any fast, or any food you eat. If you exceed what your body will use, energy/food wise, then you'll gain weight. So, it is possible that you'll gain weight when fasting. But if you do, it's not because of a lower metabolic rate, and is more because of poorly planned diet. To prevent this, it's important that you eat well-balanced nutritious foods. This will help you maintain weight, or possibly lose some if it's a shift from your normal diet. You could also combine calorie restriction with fasting, and we'll discuss this in a later chapter. Basically, if you gain weight when fasting, then it's due to diet and you'll need to watch what you eat to lose or maintain your weight.

Myth #3: Fasting is not Sustainable Long-term

There are so many diets out there that are not sustainable. What immediately comes to mind are the types of diet where you eat only one type of food, like the cabbage soup diet. These kinds of diets are not sustainable because it's easy to start craving more types of food. Your body itself will crave the nutrients it needs, while you'll get bored with that single kind of food. A lot of diets that are fad diets aren't sustainable because they often don't provide your body with the requirements it needs to function well. This results in you being hungry and craving the foods that are prohibited in those diets. Fasting isn't like fad and doesn't restrict certain types of food. So, while you might get hungry, it's unlikely you'll have any brutal cravings. This can increase the sustainability of fasting.

Also, there are so many kinds of fasting. Some of them are really easy to incorporate into your daily life, like the 14/10 fast or the 16/8 fast. With these diets, you're simply extending your fast further than your normal eight hours of sleep. Sometimes this means eating your last meal early, or your first meal late. Because these two types are simple and easy to get into, it can be easy to maintain as well. Other types of fasting can be even easier, depending on your own personality. But the reality remains that fasting can be quickly started and maintained.

Finally, a lot of people find fasting much easier to sustain than long term calorie restriction. Long-term calorie restriction is your typical, doctor approved diet. You reduce your eaten calories by a bit every day and you lose weight. However, this can be difficult to maintain because it requires you to pick and choose what you eat carefully and can restrict social eating. In a study comparing alternate day fasting and calorie restriction, the researchers found that the participants felt the fasting was easier to sustain (Alhamdan, 2016).

This has been echoed in other studies and even anecdotally. Even though hunger could be an issue with alternate day fasting, that's not always the case as participants found that their hunger on fasting days was reduced after two weeks of following the fast schedule (Klemple et al., 2010). So, fasting can be easy to start, maintain, and sustain because it doesn't restrict you.

Intermittent fasting is considered a lifestyle change. I know this is mentioned in many different diets, but with fasting, it's the easiest way to change your eating habits. It can change your health and reduce your weight. By following it in the long-term, you'll maintain all those benefits. So, fasting is and can be sustainable.

Myth #4: Fasting Causes you to Binge

This myth is based slightly on reality. It comes from how we often react when we skip a meal. We all know the feeling. You've decided to work through lunch and by the time you get home, you are dramatically dying of hunger. You go to your pantry and start gorging on anything that will fill that empty void and end hunger. When we come to, we're surrounded by the remnants of what we've eaten. It can be very surprising how much has been eaten during a moment of, what feels like, desperate hunger.

The thing that can be doubly amazing is that during this feeling of almost insatiable hunger, our bodies are sending out signals that tell us to eat, but also to stop after a certain point. Unfortunately, most of us are incapable of hearing that, "I'm full" signal from our brains when in this state. So, we overeat. By a lot. This is a typical feeling of a binge. If we get to the point where we're very hungry, we often just start eating everything available and have a hard time stopping. So yes, it's possible that you'll binge when breaking your fast with your first meal. But it doesn't have to happen, and it doesn't happen to many people. This is because people understand how their hunger works, and how to break their fast properly to prevent binging.

When breaking your fast, you want to ease into it. Depending on what type of fast you have, you may be breaking your fast after 14 hours, or after 24 hours. So it's important to slowly break your fast. Don't just start gorging on everything you see. Take a deep breath. Have some coffee or tea. Then start eating with something small. Take a short break, and then eat a little more. Listen for your "I'm full" signal from your body. Then stop eating.

A way that can also help with this feeling is to be more mindful while you eat. Mindfulness is a common term now a days, but it can be applied to eating. Mindfulness means that you make yourself become aware of the 'now' moment. What is happening right now? What are you seeing, hearing, tasting, feeling, and smelling? At this very moment where are you and how did you get there? All of this is taking a step back and focusing on this present moment. When following mindfulness, you are not just focused on one thing, but also allowing your thoughts to come and go without you evaluating them or judging yourself. But what does this have to do with eating and binging?

Mindfulness and eating can go hand in hand. Essentially, you want to look at your current present moment, but also being aware of your body's reaction as you eat. It means eating slowly, tasting each piece of food you put in your mouth, and slowly savoring it. You could focus on your five senses while you eat and say exactly what each of them is feeling. It's also about listening to your body's reaction and looking for that full signal. Being aware of our body and how we're filling up can help us ensure that we're not giving into the hunger monster.

With mindfulness in your toolkit, you can learn what the full feeling means to your body. You can learn when to slow down and to stop eating. This can take some time. We often bypass the full feeling, so don't stress yourself as it will take time for you to get used to it. It can come along much earlier than you may have felt before, but if you can remain mindful while you eat, you can reduce the likelihood of binging. Be mindful as you eat so that you're paying attention to your hunger signals. All these things can help you break your fast without binging. So, there is some truth to this myth, but it's easily managed and prevented.

Myth #5: You Can Eat Whatever You Want

With most intermittent fasting methods, you don't have to restrict your diet when you have your eating window. This isn't in all methods, just some. The myth that you can eat whatever you want comes from this unrestriction on what you're eating. Much like the myth before this one, there is some truth to this. While fasting, you still eat whatever you want, but solely in your eating window. If you want to eat fast food every single day during your eating window, then go ahead. But...it's very likely that fasting won't help you in this case. If you're eating unhealthy foods, you're likely consuming too many calories with very little nutritious value to it. This will result in you not losing weight. In fact, you might even gain weight.

If you gain weight while fasting, look at your diet. What you eat can change how the fast will affect you. You might have better insulin levels, but you may also have a worse metabolic rate, on top of weight gain. Instead of eating a pint of ice cream every day (you know you want to), try to limit yourself and eat well-balanced meals in between your pints. If you want to lose weight, make sure that your meals are very healthy. This will ensure that the fast impacts you positively.

Myth #6: You'll be Constantly Hungry

This myth is based on fear, pure and simple. We can feel insanely hungry if we just skip a meal. What if we skip 14 hours of meals! In our minds, this sounds terrifying. We think that we'll end up being hungry all the time. Well, we will probably feel some hunger, but it won't be constant. Afterall, if you're not eating for 14 hours, then yes, you're going to feel hungry. But once you eat in your eating window, you will obviously not feel hungry anymore. If you don't believe me, then look at some of the human participants in research, or really an anecdotal evidence from those who have done intermittent fasting.

In some research, when participants completed alternate day fasting, they didn't feel very hungry once they got used to the schedule (Klemple et al., 2010). Of course, this wasn't for all participants, but for many of them, their hunger was reduced. Additionally, you can look at any blog or forum about intermittent fasting, and you'll see that a lot of people talk about how their hunger pangs were reduced after fasting for a bit. Their bodies got used to the fasting schedule, and they felt less hungry during fasting periods or days. Based on this information, it's very unlikely that you'll be constantly hungry.

Chapter 3: Benefits and Risks

After spending so much time tell you what not to believe, we've now come to the chapter that will tell you the great things about intermittent fasting. There are just so many unexpected benefits of fasting, and while I'm sure you started reading this book hoping to just lose weight with fasting, you can gain so many more health benefits than just weight loss. Unfortunately, there's nothing perfect in life, and I'm sad to say that intermittent fasting isn't perfect. There are always some risks and drawbacks of fasting. We'll also cover these in this chapter.

While reading this benefits and risks, keep in mind that not everyone will react the same way. How you react to fasting isn't going to be the same as how someone else does. So, look at your health with a critical eye and consider whether the benefits will help you or whether the risks will harm you. You can also just do a trial and error fast to see how your body will react, but always do so with wisdom.

In this chapter, we'll have some of the research studies

mentioned that are about intermittent fasting. It's important to mention some of the limitations of these studies. Intermittent fasting is so recent that there isn't enough research yet on the human experience while intermittent fasting. There is some research, but not a lot. More research has been done on animals that are like humans biologically, like some apes. Some less similar animals are rodents, and there are a lot of studies on fasting with rodents. Some of these will be mentioned here and some will be human studies. But all will help explain the benefits and risks.

Benefits of Intermittent Fasting

Generally intermittent fasting has way more benefits than risks. The one everyone knows about is weight loss. But there are so many other benefits too. One of the best benefits is how intermittent fasting changes your hormone levels, so that your insulin levels are lowered. There are also some other benefits for your heart, brain, and body.

Weight loss

Weight loss it the most well-known benefit of intermittent fasting. Even this book has the word "weight loss" in the title. During intermittent fasting, it's likely that you'll lose some weight. Whether you're following the easier 14/10 method or the harder alternate day method, you're going to lose some weight. There are a couple of reasons why this is, but the biggest one is because of calorie restriction.

Calorie restriction is one of the most common methods of weight loss recommended by doctors. We've already discussed a bit of how calorie restriction works and how unplanned versus planned calorie restriction works in fasting. In simplified 14/10 fasts and ones like it, you'll have some unplanned calorie restriction which can help you with weight loss. To get the most out of calorie restriction, you would want to follow the alternate day style of fasting. This is because there's just such a massive reduction in calories on those alternate days. Alternate day fasting has been found to be equivalent to regular, doctor approved, calorie reduction in multiple studies (Alhamdan et al., 2016; Klemple et al., 2010;

Anson et al., 2003). Even better yet, because calorie reduction is interspersed with full regular meals every other day, this style of fasting is easier to stick with rather than a regular calorie restricted diet.

So, you can expect some weight loss while intermittent fasting. However, this also depends on other aspects of your lifestyle. We've talked about the importance of diet before, but we haven't talked about the importance of exercising. Doing regular exercising while intermittent fasting can also increase how much weight you lose, without losing a lot of muscle mass from the fast. You don't have to exercise heavily, but if you want to, you could go for a 30-minute walk, a bike ride or a swim. All of these can help maintain your weight loss while also maintaining your muscle mass.

The last thing to mention is that once you finish your fasting, in the case where you're not doing this for the rest of your life, you'll be less likely to regain the weight. This isn't based on a lot of research, but some people suggest that because fasting changes how you eat and your relationship with food, you don't return to your previous style of eating. Take it or leave it, but you'll still have some improvement in your weight with intermittent fasting.

Intermittent fasting can reduce insulin levels and insulin resistance. Did you know that one-third of Americans are diagnosed with pre-diabetes? That's quite a lot and is often due to our carb and sugar laden diets. So many people in the U.S. struggle with their blood sugar levels and insulin levels. Essentially, in prediabetes your blood sugar levels are consistently higher than normal, and your body tries to fix this by increasing your insulin. Insulin is what helps your body to absorb the glucose from your food to use as energy. However, when experiencing prediabetes, your cells become resistant to the insulin. This increases the cycle again, with more insulin coming into your bloodstream and more insulin resistance occurring. This can be very problematic and result in having a diagnosis of type 2 diabetes, stroke, obesity or heart disease. Intermittent fasting can help with your insulin levels and insulin resistance.

When intermittent fasting, the blood-glucose levels can be a little more controlled, insulin resistance is reduced, and insulin itself is also reduced. This is something that has been repeated in several studies. The insulin decreases because of the way the body uses the glucose from eating during the fasting period, but it also decreases because of weight loss that is also happening. In most studies, the type of fasting used to create some of the best changes in insulin levels was alternate day fasting. This makes a lot of sense, since it's also the style of fasting that results in the most weight loss.

Improved heart health is one of the benefits that needs to be better researched in humans. However, in animals intermittent fasting is very promising for improving heart health. Intermittent fasting helps improve cholesterol levels, blood pressure, and inflammation. All of which can lead to better heart health. Obviously, this is important because since there are so many things that can negatively affect heart health. So, if intermittent fasting can help reduce these things, then you'll have a lower risk of heart disease, heart attacks, and other cardiovascular problems.

There is some research that suggests intermittent fasting can help with ageing and brain health. It has to do with how your cells recuperate from cellular stress and metabolism. The research suggests that intermittent fasting can help reduce the likelihood of Alzhemiers and Parkinson's diseases (Martin et al., 2009). While this research is very promising, there hasn't been enough human research to say this. However, the promise of better brain health is something to look forward to with intermittent fasting.

Risks of Intermittent Fasting

The risks of intermittent fasting are varied. If people fast when they shouldn't (see chapter 1), then the risks of intermittent fasting can be quite severe. However, for most people intermittent fasting isn't very risky. The risks you'll run into are bingeing, malnutrition, and difficulty with maintaining the fast. We've talked about bingeing quite extensively, so we're not going to discuss it much more. Suffice it to say, bingeing while you fast risks any of the benefits from fasting you might originally have. A bigger risk is malnutrition.

Malnutrition sounds alarming, but for the most part, you can prevent this by having well-balanced meals during your eating windows. The risk of malnutrition comes especially during the kinds of fast which include very low-calorie restriction on fasting days. Fasts like this are 5:2 fasts and alternate day fasting. If you're not eating the right nutrition throughout your week, the reduction in calories plus the poor nutrition can result in some of your dietary needs not being met. This could result in more weight loss, but also more muscle loss and other issues. To prevent this risk, you can ensure that your meals are nutritious and well-balanced. Have a variety of fruits and vegetables, try different meats and seafoods, and include grains unless you're following a specific diet like the keto diet.

Associated with malnutrition is dehydration. We get a lot of our daily water intake from the food we eat. But if you're eating a reduced amount of food during your day, or no food during your day, you're going to need to drink a lot more water than you normally do. If you're not keeping track of your hydration levels, it's possible for you to drink too little. To combat this risk, ensure that you're drinking enough by keeping a hydration journal. You could also track it in an app. Set up reminders to drink water and check your urine color. Light colored urine means good hydration, so check often despite how disgusting it might be to you.

Because fasting can be difficult to start, this can be one of the risks associated with it. You're going to feel hungry during the first couple weeks of following your fasting schedule. You may even feel uncomfortable, with mood swings, different bowel movements, and sleep disruptions. All of this can lead to you struggling with starting the fasts. They can also lead you to ignore greater warning signs that you shouldn't fast. These signs include changed heart rate, feelings of weakness, and extreme fatigue. These feelings shouldn't be ignored during the start. If you feel severely uncomfortable when you start your fast, you should stop and speak with your doctor.

Chapter 4: Styles of Intermittent Fasting

Now that you've learned the basics of intermittent fasting, it's time to go into the different types. There isn't just one style of intermittent fasting. There are basic styles like fasting for a full 24 hours, but there are also other kinds that take advantage of our normal daily activities and leave us slightly less hungry. Whichever method you choose, you'll still receive some good health benefits. There are five different varieties of intermittent fasting that will be covered in this chapter: the 14/10 method, 5:2 method, 24 Hour method, Warrior Diet method, and the Alternate Day method. These five methods have been organized from easiest to hardest.

One method that won't be discussed in this chapter is the 16/8 method. It is by far one of the easiest styles of intermittent fasting to get into and to maintain in the long-term. While we won't be covering it in this book, we did write another book that goes into the 16/8 method and provides a step-by-step guide for how to follow it. If you're interested in learning more, please look at *Intermittent Fasting 16/8: The Complete Step-by-Step Guide.*

14/10 Method

The 14/10 method takes advantage of your daily schedule to add some areas of fasting. It is a type of fasting that is called Time Restricted Eating (TRE). When reading studies about intermittent fasting, you'll see this phrase used often and it is usually referring to the 16/8, 14/10, or 12/12 methods. The 14/10 method is easy to follow, and thus, is a simple way to transition into intermittent fasting. In this method, you fast for 14 hours and then eat during a 10-hour window. It may sound a little difficult, but it isn't. Considering that you'll sleep for some of your 14 hours of fasting, you won't have to fast for as long as you think.

What many people do when they follow this style, is that they extend their fast on both sides of when they go to sleep. For instance, assuming you sleep for eight hours at night, then you'll add three hours of fasting before bed, and three hours after bed. Sometimes this doesn't work for people's schedule, especially if breakfast if important to you. In cases like this, people fast for the extra 6 hours before bed and have their last meal quite early in the day.

Because there isn't a huge shift in how you eat, when you eat, this style of intermittent fasting can be quite beneficial for people. It's something that doesn't change your normal habits very much, which is appealing to many. Afterall, if something new requires a massive change, then you'll be less likely to stick with it. The convenience of the plan also means that you're not going to have a huge difference between when you normally eat and when you eat on the fast. These smaller changes mean that you're more likely to follow the fasting plan and stay motivated to complete it.

Another benefit of this style fast is that you can still make room for social eating, unlike in other plans. If you want to have dinner with your friends, then all you must do is shift your eating and fasting windows so that you can be with your friends. Since this style of fasting doesn't require a different diet, it means that you also won't have to restrict your calories while you're eating out with your friends and family. While a diet isn't a requirement, having a well-balanced meal is recommended.

5:2 Method

This method has recently become more popular. Even comedian Jimmy Kimmel follows this style of fasting, with great results. While the 14/10 method is about when you eat, the 5:2 method is about what and when you eat. This method means that you'll eat regularly for five days a week, but then have two days where you eat a drastically reduced calorie diet. While most people eat roughly 2,200 calories in a day, while you're on the 5:2 fast, you'll eat your 2,200 calories for five days, but then eat only 500-600 calories on the two fasting days.

The benefits of having the calorie restriction twice per week means that you are more likely to lose weight, even if you overeat slightly on the days when you follow your normal diet. The 5:2 diet hasn't been more heavily researched than many other kinds of intermittent fasting, but what has been researched shows some promising studies about it. While many studies are with animals as subjects, there are a few with human participants too.

In some of the studies, it is believed that the 5:2 method can reduce tumors in breast cancer and help with other physiological issues in the body. It can help improve insulin resistance and prevent cardiovascular disease. While these studies are promising, just keep in mind that many of them revolved around animals. You can find the studies in the reference page at the end of this book, if you would like to do further research.

In general, the 5:2 method can provide you with weight loss that is on par with people who reduce calories every day. However, some people find reducing calories everyday to be very restrictive. Afterall, there's only so much you can eat on a calorie restrictive diet. However, with the 5:2 method you can eat whatever you want for your eating days, and only reduce your calories on your fasting day. While you can eat whatever you want, you should still maintain a well-balanced diet. Eating only junk food won't help with your weight loss goals, if that is the reason you're choosing to fast.

While the 5:2 method can be very beneficial, some people struggle with their first few fast days. After eating 2,000 calories on day one followed by 500 calories on day two, you can feel almost uncontrollably hungry. However, many people say (anecdotally) that the hunger fades if you keep yourself distracted. Also, so long as you follow the fast for a while, you'll soon no longer feel hungry during your fast days. All of this is anecdotal of course, but it is something to consider when choosing to fast with the 5:2 method.

24 Hour

The 24-hour fast is exactly how it sounds. You simply choose to fast entirely for 24 hours. During this fast, you don't eat at all during your fasting hours, but this doesn't mean that you can't eat during the day of your fast. One-way people cope with the 24 hours of not eating is to start their fast immediately after dinner, and then stop it at the same time the next day. This way, you're still eating on both days, just with a very long time between meals. If this is confusing to you, then here's a clarification: If you finish dinner at 7pm, then that time is your fasting start time. You would continue to fast until 7pm the next day and have your first meal right after that time. This way, you're eating something still, which might help console you.

This timing can be better than if you choose to fast from the moment you wake up one morning to the moment you wake up the next morning. This is how many people first interpret the 24-hour fast, but it is incorrect. If you followed that interpretation, then you would eat dinner at 7pm, maybe have a midnight snack at 12am, fast until you wake up at 8am, and keep fasting until 8am the next day. This places you at 32-37 hours of fasting. So, if you choose to do 24 hours fasting, then really make sure you're counting the 24 hours.

This style of fasting can give you the same benefits as other kinds of intermittent fasting. It provides an overall, weekly calorie reduction, which will lead to weight loss. However, a lot of people can struggle with this kind of fast. Going without food for 24 hours is hard, and can make you feel weak and faint, with low energy levels. On the other hand, some people find it easier to handle than the 5:2 fast, because they think having even a tiny bit of food makes you start craving more. Whichever side of the fence you fall on, the 24-hour fast is still beneficial.

Besides feeling a bit hungry during your 24 hours of fasting, there is a likelihood that you'll binge more the next day because you've simply not had anything the day before. Even if you binge a bit, it's unlikely that you'll eat a full day's worth of extra calories. So, you'll still have a weekly calorie reduction.

The Warrior Diet

The Warrior Diet is labelled as a diet, but it's typically a style of intermittent fasting. The Warrior Diet is called such because it's believed to follow the eating habits of ancient warriors. It's based on the belief that warriors would eat very little during the day and then overeat at night in a 'feast.' Essentially, this leads to a 20:4 fast, with 20 hours of fasting, and four hours of eating. Having only four hours to eat can be very difficult for people, especially if you're supposed to overeat. For many of us, having a heavy meal at nighttime can interrupt our sleep habits and can make us feel ill. For others, having to eat so much after a long fast can lead to some gastric distress. So, the Warrior Diet has some areas that people may struggle with.

What you eat is just as important as when you eat during this fast. It's recommended you eat unprocessed foods, with a lot of raw vegetables and fruits. During your 20 hours of fasting, you can eat tiny amounts of fruit and vegetables, but some people will find it difficult to sustain their day on this. With the change in diet and eating time, the Warrior Diet will supposedly cause a clearer mind and better cellular repair. This is possible, since eating less processed food can result in ketosis which helps with cellular repair, and there is some research supporting intermittent fasting for improved brain function. While there isn't a lot of research on the Warrior Diet itself, because it is technically a type of intermittent fasting, some of the research found could carry over to the Warrior Diet. So, it's possible it will lead to weight loss but it's also possible that it won't. There simply isn't enough research out there to promote a 20:4 fast.

The Warrior Diet might work in theory, but it will depend on the type of person who is following it. If you have a lot of dedication, motivation, and a good understanding of nutrition, you could do very well with the Warrior Diet. However, if you're leaving a carbohydrate heavy diet, with three meals a day, the Warrior Diet can be a severe change which can reduce your motivation to continue. Beyond this, with only a four-hour eating window, it can be difficult to do social eating activities, like having brunch, or eating out with your co-workers for lunch. This can strain the motivation and sustainability of those who are trying to follow the diet. This is why it's one of the harder versions of intermittent fasting to follow.

Alternate Day

Alternate Day fasting is like an extended version of the 5:2 method. There's actually a lot of research that supports alternate day fasting, and it's considered to be really good for reducing belly fat in people who are very obese. Even if weight is maintained, there's a good chance that alternate day fasting can lead to better health overall. It can reduce insulin levels and insulin resistance and can help the brain handle cell stress (Anson et al., 2003). There are a lot of studies about it, but as mentioned before, some of these studies are animal studies. However, they provide some promising implications for how alternate day fasting can help humans.

In this fast, you are fasting every other day, and eating your regular portions on your off days. This means that you have an overall reduced calorie load during the week. This is similar to a regular calorie reduction diet, where calories are reduced everyday. So, the weekly calorie restriction can be the same in both the fast and the diet. However, people generally find alternate day fasting easier to follow than calorie restricted diets. There are some people who dislike the alternate day fast because it can be very difficult to go hungry during the fasting days. This hunger doesn't always get easier as the weeks go on. This can strain people's motivation to continue the fast. Some people combat this by eating a reduced calorie meal on fasting days. In this case, this adaptation makes the alternate day fast like the 5:2 fast, with just extra days of fasting.

Because there is a significant calorie reduction, it's important that the meals you eat are nutritious. You don't want to be undernourished while following this fast. Additionally, if you're already at a healthy weight, this fast may make you lose weight that you can't afford to lose. So be careful when approaching this fast. However, if you are very overweight, then this fast can help you. Just work with your doctor to figure out if this fast will be of benefit to you. As mentioned earlier, there is significant research associated with alternate day fasting, and a lot of it is positive. So, this style of fasting can bring you significant benefits.

To conclude this chapter, there are several different options for following an intermittent fast. You should choose the fasting method that works for you and your lifestyle. If you're a very social eater, then choose a fast like the 14:10 fast or perhaps the 5:2 fast. If you're very determined, have great discipline, and can maintain motivation, then choose a fast like the 24-hour, alternate day, or the Warrior Diet. Either way, you'll likely get some benefits from these fast choices. But with benefits, always comes risks. These fasts all have some risks associated and it's important to know them before choosing to follow intermittent fasting. In the next chapter, we'll be discussing the benefits of fasting in general, and explore the risks associated with fasting.

Chapter 5: Transitioning into Intermittent Fasting

Now we get into the fine print of intermittent fasting. You've learned all the basics of intermittent fasting in general, but it's time to learn how to start your fasts. In this chapter, we'll look at transitioning schedules for each kind of fast. Use the schedules to help you determine which fasts will work for you and which ones are not going to work for your lifestyle.

One recommendation I have for you is to track your fast by maintaining a journal. Your journal can help you with your schedule, but also can be a consistent record of which styles have worked for you, which have not, and where you are struggling with the fasts. When you have your journal set up, start by including your chosen fasting schedule and why you've chosen that one. Also add your goals to the journal and write down what works and doesn't for you. Keep it regularly updated and you'll have a beautiful record of your fasting journey.

Before looking at our schedules, there are some things to keep in mind.

- Each of the schedules below will give you some variation of how to start and transition into them. So, when you choose your schedule, you'll have plenty of options to choose from. However, if you don't find a schedule that works for you, then create your own! Each one is personal.

- The schedules don't have to be permanent. Don't feel like you're committed to one type of schedule simply because you've already been using it for several weeks. If it's not working, change it up and choose a different schedule. And if you want to eat out during your fasting window, then just shift your fasting and eating time to fit your social schedule. This isn't an inseparable marriage. Simply choose and adapt your schedule to fit you and don't feel any guilt about changing them as you go along.

- Ideally, you want to transition slowly. So, each schedule will demonstrate a slow transition into the fast. If you don't want to go slow, that's your choice. But going slow will help you ease into the fast and reduce the likelihood of feeling those negative emotions we discussed before. Each of these schedules shows a transition period of two weeks before you're fully following the schedule.

Transitioning into 14:10

When transitioning into the 14:10 schedule, you have a variety of options. You can choose to have an early eating schedule, where your first meal is very early in the morning. You could follow the mid-day eating schedule, or you could follow the late day eating schedule. Choose the one that fits your lifestyle. If you're a shift worker, the late day eating schedule might work best for you. If you're an early morning person, then that schedule will be your best bet. So, choose the one that fits you best.

Early Eating Schedule

If you want to follow your body's natural rhythm of being more active during the early morning, then this is the schedule for you. It's also great because it gives you a decent time in the evening where you'll be without food, which can help you when you sleep. In this schedule, you'll start eating at 7am and end at 5pm. This is a slow transition, so it's a one hour transition every couple of days over the course of two weeks.

Time	Day 1-3	Day 4-6	Day 7-9	Day 10-12
7 A.M.	Wake up Eat	Wake up Eat	Wake up Eat	Wake up Eat
9 A.M.	Eat	Eat	Eat	Eat
11 A.M.	Eat	Eat	Eat	Eat
1 P.M.	Eat	Eat	Eat	Eat
3 P.M.	Snack	Eat	Eat	Eat
5 P.M.	Eat	Eat	Eat	Eat before 5

7 P.M.	Eat	Eat	Fast	Fast
9 P.M.	Eat	Fast	Fast	Fast
10 P.M.-	Sleep/ Fast	Sleep/ Fast	Sleep/ Fast	Sleep/ Fast

Once you've transitioned into the fast, here is what your week will look like:

Time	12 A.M. - 7 A.M.	7 am	12 P.M.	4 P.M.	5 P.M. - 12 A.M.
Monday - Sunday	Fast/sleep	Breakfast	Large meal	Last meal, finished by 5 P.M.	Fast/Sleep

Mid-day Eating Schedule

The mid-day eating schedule works for people who aren't morning people. It's also something that you can follow on the weekends, if you want a later start to your day. This schedule is also great because you can have more of a social life than in the early eating schedule. After all, most people eat dinner out socially usually after 5pm. Again, this schedule is a transition over the course of a couple of weeks. This may help reduce your feelings of discomfort as you transition. In this schedule, you start eating at 10am and finish your last meal by 8pm.

Time	Day 1-3	Day 4-6	Day 7-9	Day 10-12
6 A.M.	Sleep/Eat	Sleep/ Fast	Sleep/ Fast	Sleep/ Fast
8 A.M.	Eat	Eat	Fast	Fast

10 A.M.	Eat	Eat	Eat	Eat
12 P.M.	Eat	Eat	Eat	
2 P.M.	Snack	Snack		Eat
4 P.M.	Eat	Eat	Eat	Eat
6 P.M.	Eat	Eat	Eat	
8 P.M.	Eat	Eat	Eat	Eat before 8
10 P.M. -	Sleep/Fast	Sleep/Fast	Sleep/Fast	Sleep/Fast

Once you've transitioned into the fast, here is what your week will look like:

Time	12 A.M. - 7 A.M.	10 A.M.	2 P.M.	7 P.M.	8 P.M. - 12 A.M.
Monday - Sunday	Fast/sleep	Breakfast	Large meal	Last meal, finished by 8 P.M.	Fast/Sleep

Evening Eating Schedule

Many people have difficulty eating late at night. However, if you're a night owl and want to have later meals, this schedule is for you. There are some things to notice about this schedule. First is that our bodies don't normally metabolize food efficiently at night. So, you may have difficulty sleeping if you eat too late, and you won't have the same benefits with glucose as you would by eating early in the day. However, this schedule is perfect if you plan on partying with your friends late at night, or if you work unconventional hours. Just like before, this fast transitions over the course of a couple weeks. Your eating window starts at 2pm and ends at 12am.

Time	Day 1-3	Day 4-6	Day 7-9	Day 10-12
12 A.M - 6 A.M.	Sleep/ Fast	Sleep/ Fast	Sleep/ Fast	Sleep/ Fast
8 A.M.	Eat	Fast	Fast	Fast
10 A.M.	Eat	Eat	Fast	Fast
12 P.M.	Eat	Eat	Eat	Fast
2 P.M.	Snack	Eat	Eat	Eat

4 P.M.	Eat	Eat	Snack	Eat
6 P.M.	Eat	Snack	Eat	Eat
8 P.M.	Eat	Eat	Eat	Eat
10 P.M.	Eat	Eat	Eat	Eat
12 A.M.	Eat	Eat	Eat	Eat before midnight

Once you've transitioned into the fast, here is what your week will look like:

Time	12 A.M. - 8 A.M.	8 A.M. - 2.P.M.	2 P.M.	7 P.M.	11 P.M. - 12 A.M.

Monday - Sunday	Fast/sleep	Fast	Breakfast	Large meal	Last meal, finished by midnight

With these three schedules, you have a variety of opportunities to fast following the 14/10 method. Make sure that you take the time to make these schedules yours. Adapt them to your schedule and your family situation. You can also shift your schedule over a couple of days. If the early morning schedule appeals to you, but you like having dinner out with friends every Friday night, then you may choose to shift your eating windows for the weekend. This way you're still fasting for 14 hours and eating within a 10-hour window.

Transitioning into 5:2

The 5:2 schedule is different from the 14/10 schedule. It doesn't require a daily fast, but instead requires two days of fasting within the week. During those two days, you'll eat just 500-600 calories for that day. In this section, we'll look at two possible schedules for your 5:2 fast. The first schedule is one where you fast on Mondays and Thursdays. The second option is a fast on Wednesdays and Saturdays. If you choose to create your own schedule, make sure that you have a couple of days between each fasting day. Don't fast for Saturday and Sunday. That's 48 hours with limited calories and isn't good for your body. You'll also feel incredibly hungry by the time you eat on Monday. So, if you are following your own schedule, make sure you have a couple of days between each fasting day.

Monday and Thursday fasting days

This schedule is perfect for those who are comfortable being at work without much food. For some of us, this doesn't work. However, if you feel very comfortable with it, then this schedule will work for you. Remember that during your fasting days, you can eat 500-600 calories. During your eating days, you can eat what you want, but try not to overeat or you'll undo the good you did during your fast. This schedule will transition you over the course of a couple of weeks.

Week 1

Time	Mon	Tue	Wed	Thurs	Fri	Sat	Sun
8 A.M.	Fast	Eat all day	Eat all day	Fast	Eat all day	Eat all day	Eat all day
12 P.M.	Eat 800 calories	Eat	Eat	Eat 600 calories	Eat	Eat	Eat
4 P.M.		Eat	Eat		Eat	Eat	Eat

8 P.M.	Eat 400 calories	Eat	Eat	Eat 400 calories	Eat	Eat	Eat
10 P.M.	Sleep / Fast	Sleep/ Fast	Sleep/ Fast	Sleep / Fast	Eat	Eat	Eat
12 P.M	Sleep / Fast	Sleep/ Fast	Sleep/ Fast	Sleep / Fast	Sleep/ Fast	Sleep/ Fast	Sleep/ Fast

Week 2

Time	Mon	Tue	Wed	Thurs	Fri	Sat	Sun
8 A.	Fast	Eat all	Eat all	Fast	Eat all	Eat all	Eat all

M.		day	day		day	day	day
12 P.M.	Eat 400 calories	Eat	Eat	Eat 400 calories	Eat	Eat	Eat
4 P.M.	Fast	Eat	Eat	Fast	Eat	Eat	Eat
8 P.M.	Eat 400 calories	Eat	Eat	Eat 300 calories	Eat	Eat	Eat
10 P.M.	Sleep / Fast	Sleep/ Fast	Sleep/ Fast	Sleep / Fast	Eat	Eat	Eat
12	Sleep	Slee	Slee	Sleep	Slee	Slee	Slee

P.M	/	p/	p/	/	p/	p/	p/
	Fast	Fast	Fast	Fast	Fast	Fast	Fast

You can see in this schedule; you're increasing your fasting time from week one to week two on your fasting days. There's also a mid-day fast within week two. When you fully transition into your fast, your week will look like this:

Mon	Tue	Wed	Thur	Friday	Sat	Sun
Fast day: Eat 500-600 calories through the day,	Eating day: Eat what you want, but don't overeat.	Eating day	Fast day: Eat 500-600 calories through the day,	Eating day: Eat what you want, but don't overeat.	Eating day	Eating day

or eat one large meal	Break your fast carefully		or eat one large meal	Break your fast carefully		

In the schedule above, you should have noticed the additional note to break your fast carefully. Because you'll be breaking your fast after a day with very low calories, you want to break it slowly. Start your breakfast with something that is light, not too heavy, and not something sugary. If you don't, you may feel some gastric upset and nausea. So, break your fast with some tea or bone broth, have a bit of yogurt and nuts, or something else light for you. Once you break your fast, you can eat normally throughout the day. There's more about breaking your fast in the section on transitioning into the 24 hours fast.

Wednesday and Saturday fasting days

This schedule works well for those who want to fast over a weekend day. This can be great if you tend to feel faint or very hungry when fasting. It can also be less distracting than if you're sitting at work watching everyone eat donuts and coffee while you're fasting. This schedule might not work for you if you're a very social eater over the weekends. So, take that into consideration before choosing this schedule.

Week 1

Time	Mon	Tue	Wed	Thurs	Fri	Sat	Sun
8 A.M.	Eat all day	Eat all day	Fast	Eat all day	Eat all day	Fast	Eat all day
12 P.M.	Eat	Eat	Eat 800 calori	Eat	Eat	Eat 600 calori	Eat

			es			es	
4 P.M.	Eat	Eat	Eat	Eat	Eat	Eat	Eat
8 P.M.	Eat	Eat	Eat 400 calories	Eat	Eat	Eat 400 calories	Eat
10 P.M.	Sleep/ Fast	Sleep/ Fast	Sleep/ Fast	Sleep/ Fast	Eat		Eat
12 P.M	Sleep/ Fast	Sleep/ Fast	Sleep/ Fast	Sleep/ Fast	Sleep/ Fast	Sleep/ Fast	Sleep/ Fast

Week 2

Time	Mon	Tue	Wed	Thurs	Fri	Sat	Sun
8 A.M.	Eat all day	Eat all day	Fast	Eat all day	Eat all day	Fast	Eat all day
12 P.M.	Eat	Eat	Eat 400 calories	Eat	Eat	Eat 400 calories	Eat
4 P.M.	Eat	Eat	Fast	Eat	Eat	Fast	Eat
8 P.M.	Eat	Eat	Eat 400 calories	Eat	Eat	Eat 300 calories	Eat
10	Slee	Slee	Sleep	Slee	Eat	Fast	Eat

P.M.	p/ Fast	p/ Fast	/ Fast	p/ Fast			
12 P.M	Slee p/ Fast	Slee p/ Fast	Sleep / Fast	Slee p/ Fast	Slee p/ Fast	Sleep / Fast	Slee p/ Fast

When you fully transition into your fast, your week will look like this:

Mon	Tue	Wed	Thur	Friday	Sat	Sun
Eating day	Eating day	Fast day: Eat 500-600 calories	Eating day: Eat what you want, but	Eating day	Fast day: Eat 500-600 calories	Eating day: Eat what you want, but

		through the day, or eat one large meal	don't overeat. Break your fast carefully		through the day, or eat one large meal	don't overeat. Break your fast carefully

In both these fasting plans, you'll notice that there are some recommendations for how many calories to eat on your fasting days as you transition. These are recommendations, with the hope that it will be easier to do the full fast in week three. However, shifting to such few calories can be a little jarring. So, if you need to take it slower, go ahead! Do whatever help your body adjust to the fast best. These plans put 'breakfast' as the largest meal and it's the one that shifts to fewer and fewer calories for the fasting days. This is because it's better to have a larger meal in the morning than in the evening.

For your fasting days, you can choose to eat your 500-

600 calories all in one meal, or you may choose to break it up over a couple meals/snacks. In these plans we put them as two meals, but it can also be an all-day grazing situation. You could just snack on fruits and vegetables throughout the day, with some protein interspersed. This can help you feel fuller throughout your day, rather than just eating one large meal. However, you want to choose what you'll do based on your situation. We'll discuss some options for meals in a later chapter.

Transitioning into 24 Hour Fast

This fast is very flexible, as there's no requirement for which day you choose to fast. The only thing to keep in mind is that you don't want to fast two days in a row. Keep it at just 24 hours, and no longer. This is to ensure that you're not starting your body's starvation response with further fasting.

For this fast style, there is only one example schedule. This is just to give you an idea of how to time your 24 hours, so you still have a meal everyday, while still having a 24-hour window where you're not eating. In this schedule, the fasting days are on Saturday and Tuesday. Because there isn't a set day requirement for this fast, you could choose just to fast one day, or two days in the week. If you want to fast three days, that's moving into the alternate day fasting, which we'll talk about later in this chapter.

Here is your schedule into 24 hours fasting. There isn't a transitioning period for this one, since when you choose to fast is completely random.

Time	Mon	Tues	Wed	Thur	Fri	Sat	Sun
12 A.M -6 A.M.	Sleep / Fast	Sleep / Fast	Sleep / Fast	Sleep / Fast	Sleep / Fast	Sleep / Fast	Sleep / Fast

8 A.M.	Eat all day	Eat	Fast	Eat all day	Eat	Fast	Eat all day
10 A.M.	Eat	Finish eating by 12. P.M.	Fast	Eat	Eat	Fast	Eat
12 P.M.	Eat	Fast	Break Fast	Eat	Eat	Fast	Eat
2 P.M.	Eat	Fast	Eat	Eat	Eat	Fast	Eat
4 P.M.	Eat	Fast	Eat	Eat	Eat	Fast	Eat

6 P.M.	Eat	Fast	Eat	Eat	Finish eating by 8 P.M.	Fast	Eat
8 P.M.	Eat	Fast	Eat	Eat	Fast	Break Fast	Eat
10 P.M.	Eat	Fast	Eat	Eat	Fast	Eat	Eat

For this kind of fast, choose to fast on the days when you won't need to do a lot of physical work. If your job if physically demanding, then fast on weekends or days when you won't work. If you just like working out a lot, then on your fasting days, you'll want to take it easy or skip all together. Whatever you do, if you decide to exercise while on this fast, make sure it's right before you break your fast. You want to eat a good mix of protein and fiber after exercising to help your muscles recover.

With a 24 hour fast, it's very important that you maintain your hydration levels. Have water, tea, and black coffee during your fast. This will help with your hunger, but also help you stay hydrated. Becoming dehydrated will cause you some damage, especially because you're not getting your hydration from food. So, keep drinking liquids throughout your day, and regularly check your hydration.

In this fast and in other 24-hour style fasts, you will want to be careful with how you break your fast.

What to Eat to Break your Fast

Once you've survived your 24 hours fast, it's time to eat again. You're going to feel hungry. There's no way around it but you might feel intensely hungry. The last thing you want to do is gorge yourself on all the food. It's possible it will all just right back up if you do so, and you'll also lose some of the benefits you received from the fast in the first place. To prevent difficulty with eating again, it's important to take things slow as you break your fast.

Start by eating a little snack such as some blueberries. Starting with a liquid like water, tea, or coffee can be a great option. Another option is to have bone broth. This will help you feel fuller, but also provide you with some good nutrients for starting your eating window. After having some liquids and a small snack, 10 minutes later eat something a bit more substantial.

You're going to want to change your food type for breaking your fast. While a bacon burger will be so tempting, it's not the best choice to break your fast. It's way too heavy, too fatty, and too much for your first meal. It can make you feel bloated, have indigestion, or make you sick to your stomach. So, if you're desperate for that burger, eat it later, long after you've broken your fast. Instead of a burger, have some light proteins and fibers. Choose some fruit that aren't going to spike your blood-sugar, like raspberries, and eat them with some yogurt. Add some sunflower or flax seeds to your yogurt for added nutrition.

Some people have a lot of difficulty with eating something sugary or full of carbs after a fast. It can cause you to feel bloated and miserable. It spikes your blood sugar very quickly after a period of having lower blood-sugar levels because of your fast. This can be jarring and result in some negative physical responses. However, some people are really used to eating sweetened cereal for breakfast or even PopTarts. If you are desperate for your oatmeal in the morning after a fast, then go ahead and eat some. Check how your body feels while and after eating. This can give you a good idea for how you respond to eating these foods after a long fast. If you find that you feel miserable, then you know to avoid those foods when breaking your fast. If you feel fine, then go ahead and stick with your normal routine.

Transitioning into the Warrior Diet

This section is more about a 20:4 intermittent fast, rather than the warrior diet itself. The warrior diet has its own transitioning recommendations, which may or may not work for everyone. It can be intense, requiring significant diet changes while also changing when you eat — all of which take place at the same time and right at the beginning of the diet. So, this can be difficult to start. For this reason, this section will talk about how to transition into a 20:4 fasting schedule over the course of a couple weeks.

Like we did for the 14:10 fast, we'll provide you with some different fasting schedules that might fit your lifestyle. Once you've transitioned, you'll have a 20-hour fasting window.

Early eating schedule

This schedule is perfect if you don't want to skip breakfast. In fact, there are a lot of people that say you shouldn't skip breakfast at all. This is partially because of your circadian rhythm. Your body is more primed to activity in the morning than in the evening. So, eating your meals in the morning can have the most benefit to you. By following the early morning schedule, you won't be going to bed on a full stomach. Sleeping with so much digestion happening can be nightmare inducing. Literally. But it can also cause you to have a restless sleep, have less energy in the morning, and just in general feel terrible. So, the early morning eating schedule is perfect for those who want to avoid these difficulties. This fasting schedule opens the eating window at 7am and ends the eating window at 11am

Here is your schedule for the 20 hours fast:

Time	Day 1-3	Day 4-6	Day 7-9	Day 10-12
7 A.M.	Wake up Eat	Wake up Eat	Wake up Eat	Wake up Eat
9 A.M.	Eat	Eat	Eat	Eat
11 A.M.	Eat	Eat	Eat	Eat before 11

1 P.M.	Eat	Eat	Eat	Fast
3 P.M.	Snack	Eat	Fast	Fast
5 P.M.	Eat	Eat	Fast	Fast
7 P.M.	Eat	Fast	Fast	Fast
9 P.M.	Fast	Fast	Fast	Fast
10 P.M.-	Sleep/ Fast	Sleep/ Fast	Sleep/ Fast	Sleep/ Fast

As you can see in this schedule, it's a very significant change every three days. This should help you shift into your 20 hours of fasting, but if you're finding it difficult, then go slower before going into the 20 hours.

Once you've transitioned into the fast, you'll have a weekly schedule that looks like this:

Time	12 A.M. - 6 A.M.	7 A.M.	10 A.M.	11 A.M.	10 P.M. -
Monday - Sunday	Fast/sleep	Breakfast	Last meal, finished by 11 A.M.	Fast	Fast/sleep

This schedule can put a strain on your social eating. If you want to eat out with friends, you can adjust your eating window, but don't do a drastic adjustment. If you abruptly change your eating window, then it's possible that you'll have more than 24 hours of fasting and this can be very jarring if you're not prepared for it.

Mid-day eating schedule

This fasting window is perfect for those who are comfortable with eating a lot during work. It's also a good window if you want to have social lunches to eat with your friends and family. Because this window is still early in the day, you'll avoid the difficulties with late night eating mentioned in the first schedule. This fasting schedule opens your eating window at 11am and closes it at 3pm.

Here is your fasting schedule for the midday eating window:

Time	Day 1-3	Day 4-6	Day 7-9	Day 10-12
6 A.M.	Sleep/ Fast	Sleep/ Fast	Sleep/ Fast	Sleep/ Fast
9 A.M.	Eat	Eat	Fast	Fast
11 A.M.	Eat	Eat	Eat	Eat
1 P.M.	Eat	Eat	Eat	Eat
3 P.M.	Snack	Snack	Eat	Eat

				before 3
5 P.M.	Eat	Eat	Eat	Fast
7 P.M.	Eat	Eat	Fast	Fast
9 P.M.	Eat	Fast	Fast	Fast
10 P.M.-	Sleep/ Fast	Sleep/ Fast	Sleep/ Fast	Sleep/ Fast

Once you've transitioned into your fast, you'll have a weekly schedule that looks like this:

Time	12 A.M. - 6 A.M.	7 A.M. -11 A.M.	11 A.M.	3 P.M.	10 P.M. -
Monday -	Fast/sleep	Fast	Break fast	Last meal,	Fast/sleep

Sunday				finished by 3 P.M.	

Evening eating schedule

This schedule is perfect if you do a lot of social eating and want to be able to eat with your friends and family at nighttime. The downside to this schedule is that it ends late enough that you may experience some discomfort while you sleep. Many people have nightmares if they eat before bed, especially if they eat a lot. You may also have a very restless sleep. If you stay up all night, then this fast will work for you. In this schedule, your eating window opens at 6pm and closes at 10pm

Here is your fasting schedule for late evening meals:

Time	Day 1-3	Day 4-6	Day 7-9	Day 10-12
6 A.M.	Sleep/ Fast	Sleep/ Fast	Sleep/ Fast	Sleep/ Fast
8 A.M.	Fast	Fast	Fast	Fast
10 A.M.	Eat	Fast	Fast	Fast
12 P.M.	Eat	Eat	Fast	Fast
2 P.M.	Snack	Eat	Eat	Fast
4 P.M.	Eat	Eat	Eat	Fast
6 P.M.	Eat	Eat	Eat	Eat
8 P.M.	Eat	Eat	Eat	Eat
10 P.M.	Eat	Eat	Eat	Eat before 10

				P.M.
11 P.M. -	Sleep/ Fast	Sleep/ Fast	Sleep/ Fast	Sleep/ Fast

Once you've transitioned into your fast, you'll have a weekly schedule that looks like this:

Time	12 A.M. - 6 A.M.	7 A.M.- 12 P.M.	12 P.M.- 6 P.M.	10 P.M.	10 P.M. -
Monday - Sunday	Fast/sleep	Fast	Fast	Break fast	Last meal, finished by 10 P.M.

While the warrior diet is a kind of intermittent fasting,

it's very difficult to follow and not recommended for most people. You'll need to eat a lot during those four hours to maintain your nutrition, and this can be quite difficult. Eating 2,000 calories within four hours is nearly impossible, so you'll have significant calorie reductions during your day. You need to ensure you eat at minimum, 1300 calories during your eating windows to help you stay healthy. Each of your meals also must be nutritious and well-balanced. If you only eat food without a lot of nutrients, but with a lot of calories, you'll end up not having enough nutrients in your diet.

During your fasting window, the official warrior diet recommends you have liquids like broth, juice, water, and vegetable juice. They also recommend eating some dairy during the fasting window. Dairy like hard boiled eggs is allowed during the fasting period. This might make it a bit easier to follow the rest of the schedule. It will also help ease your hunger.

If you want to try this type of fast, take your time and pay close attention to your body. Check-in with yourself regularly. If you find that people are becoming increasingly annoying and irritating to you, and that the hunger never ends, then this fast is not for you. Ease back into a simpler 14:10 fast or 16:8 fast.

Transitioning into Alternate Day Fasting

Alternate day fasting is the kind of fast that has the most research associated and can lead to the most gains with fasting. So, it's easy to see how it can be a very popular choice. Even though it's beneficial, it's also hard to follow. It is a 24-hour style of fast, but it happens every other day instead of just once or twice a week. The transition into this will be like the 24 hours fast. There isn't going to be a huge transition period. You just must dive in. You'll have a meal every day, but during your fasting window, you won't have any meals. This is the traditional way to do alternate day fasting. If this is too difficult for you, you could add 500 calories to your fasting days, like you would for the 5:2 fasting method.

Here is one possible fasting schedule with alternate day fasting:

Time	Mon	Tues	Wed	Thur	Fri	Sat	Sun	Monday
12 A.M. - 6 A.M.	Sleep/ Fast	Sleep/ Fast	Sleep/ Fast	Sleep/ Fast	Sleep/ Fast	Sleep/ Fast	Sleep/ Fast	Sleep/ Fast
8 A.M.	Eat	Fast	Eat all day	Eat	Fast	Eat all day	Eat	Fast
10 A.M.	Eat	Fast	Eat	Eat	Fast	Eat	Eat	Fast
12 P.M.	Eat	Fast	Eat	Eat	Fast	Eat	Eat	Fast

2 P. M.	Eat	Fast	Eat	Eat	Fast	Eat	Eat	Fast
4 P. M.	Eat	Fast	Eat	Eat	Fast	Eat	Eat	Fast
6 P. M.	Finish eating by 8 P.M.	Fast	Eat	Finish eating by 8 P.M.	Fast	Eat	Finish eating by 8 P.M.	Fast
8 P. M.	Fast	Break Fast	Eat	Fast	Break Fast	Eat	Fast	Break Fast
10 P.	Fast	Eat	Eat	Fast	Eat	Eat	Fast	Eat

M.							

In this schedule, you have some days without any fasting at all, but each day also has an eating window. This can be helpful if you struggle with having no food at all during the day. You can see how the next week starts on the opposite schedule. The whole point is to alternate days for eating and fasting, so each week will be a little different.

If you want to follow a schedule that looks more like an alternate day one, then you can follow this schedule:

Time	Mon	Tues	Wed	Thur	Fri	Sat	Sun	Monday
12 A.M - 6	Sleep/ Fast	Sleep/ Fast	Sleep/ Fast	Sleep/ Fast	Sleep/ Fast	Sleep/ Fast	Sleep/ Fast	Sleep/ Fast

A. M.								
8 A. M.	Eat all day	Fast all day	Eat all day	Fast all day	Eat all day	Fast all day	Eat all day	Fast all day
10 A. M.	Eat	Fast	Eat	Fast	Eat	Fast	Eat	Fast
12 P. M.	Eat	Fast	Eat	Fast	Eat	Fast	Eat	Fast
2 ' P. M.	Eat	Fast	Eat	Fast	Eat	Fast	Eat	Fast
4 P. M.	Eat	Fast	Eat	Fast	Eat	Fast	Eat	Fast

6 P. M.	Eat	Fast	Eat	Fast	Eat	Fast	Eat	Fast
8 P. M.	Eat	Fast	Eat	Fast	Eat	Fast	Eat	Fast
10 P. M.	Eat	Fast	Eat	Fast	Eat	Fast	Eat	Fast

This schedule is not recommended unless you're really determined. You'll see that you are already fasting while you're asleep and continue your fast into the day until the next morning. This can put you close to a 32 hour fast, so it's recommended that you follow the first alternate day schedule, and not the second. However, if you're determined to follow this kind of schedule, then choose to eat 500-600 calories on your fasting days. This can help you deal with the hunger during your fast.

Hopefully, with all these scheduling options, you'll be able to find a type of intermittent fasting that works for you. If you haven't, that's okay! Just adjust one of these schedules to better fit your life. Try not to fast beyond 24 hours at a time, but if you choose to extend your fast, then ensure you eat a small meal to help carry you over your fast. In the next chapter, we will explore some possible meal plans for intermittent fasting.

Chapter 6: Intermittent Fasting and Your Diet

We've talked a lot about the why, how, and when of intermittent fasting. Let's now look at your diet and how it can help you with fasting. There are some diets that are specific to intermittent fasts. For example, the 5:2 method and alternate day fasting both have the option of having small, calorie restricted meals during your fasting days. Most other fasts simply require you to have no food during the fasting window, and during the eating window, eating well balanced meals. The Warrior Diet recommends following a Paleo style diet to bet the most benefits from it. We'll cover all these diet options for fasting. Just remember to eat what works for you.

If you don't want to change your diet, you don't have to. Afterall, intermittent fasting isn't a diet, so you don't have to change if you don't want to. However, if you don't currently have a good diet, a change to a healthier one will help you, with or without intermittent fasting. So, we'll cover some well-balanced meals and nutrition for regular eating without restriction.

5:2 Method and Alternate Day: Calorie Restriction

In the 5:2 method and some alternate day methods, you can eat a restricted diet of 500-600 calories during your fasting window. This helps to curb hunger, and reduce your calorie intake over the course of a week. Your reduction in calories can help with putting your body in ketosis to burn more fat and can also result in more weight loss in comparison to fasting alone. With these two methods, you're getting the best of both worlds and some of the best health benefits of intermittent fasting.

A reduction from 2,000 calories a day to 600 calories can feel quite drastic. So long as you are eating your regular amount of food during your eating days, you'll be okay nutrition and health wise. To get the most out of the calorie reduction, eat a combination of protein and fiber. These two food kinds can help reduce your hunger and keep you fuller, longer.

Depending on how you want to eat throughout your day, your meals are going to vary. Some people divide their allotted calories between two meals. Some people eat one large meal with all the calories for their day in it. Some people simply snack on a variety of low-calorie foods throughout the day. Let's explore some meal types that you could have with calorie restriction. The meals mentioned here will also mention their calories so you can determine how much to eat. You can also use websites and apps to give you more recipe suggestions. Whatever you choose to eat, you need to take the time to either follow the recipe precisely or weigh out your food. This way, you'll have a precise measurement of how many calories you're eating. If you choose to snack throughout the day, we'll provide some snacking options.

It's critically important that you eat at least 1,800 calories on your eating days. This is to ensure that you have enough nutrition to last both your eating day, and your fasting days. You don't want to put too much stress on your body and make it think that you're starving yourself. If you're worried about your diet, talk to a nutritionist to ensure you're eating enough, and getting good nutrients from your meals.

During your fasting window, you could eat 600 calories of marshmallows, but they're not going to provide you with the nutrients you need. So, the ideas mentioned here for your diet contain a good mix of light proteins, fruits, vegetables, and low-fat dairy. There are also a lot of egg recipes, because eggs are amazing, and healthy.

Breakfast ideas

There are a lot of foods out there that are going to provide you with a filling meal, with little calories. These include vegetables and eggs. For breakfast, you want to mix some protein with fiber, and this works perfectly with vegetables and eggs, or fruit and yogurt. The meals in this section are all 300 calories or less. You can follow these ideas to help you choose good breakfast options. If they're not filling enough, add vegetables or fruit that are low in calories. Here are our breakfast recommendations, all for under 300 calories:

- An English muffin with cream cheese and spinach. Add some salt and red pepper to spice it up. Follow the regular serving size of cream cheese to keep the calories low.

- One apple, sliced up, and peanut butter. An apple is about 120 calories, so adjust the peanut butter amount to make up 300 calories.

- Vegetables, egg, and feta cheese frittata. Choose a low-fat variety of cheese to reduce calories. Many vegetables like zucchini are low in calories, so you could probably use a quarter zucchini and one egg per serving in the frittata.

- One cup of whole-grain cereal, with one cup of milk and fruit on the side. Choosing a whole grain cereal will help get you some good fiber. The milk is your protein.

- Oatmeal with fruit is another tasty and wholesome option. If you want to add some sugar to it, then adjust the other calories in the meal. You can also make your oatmeal with water or milk. Just adjust to accommodate your calorie intake accordingly.

- Two scrambled eggs with one piece of whole grain toast. Add some butter to your toast but check your portion size to keep the calories low. Margarine isn't recommended because it's not a healthy fat and doesn't provide you any health benefits.

- One slice of whole grain bread with peanut butter and topped with sliced bananas.

While you eat these meals, or any other meals you choose, make sure that you keep a record of how your body reacts to these meals. Do they help alleviate your hunger during a longer fast? Do they make you feel uncomfortable? Just be mindful of what you eat and how it makes you feel while eating these very low-calorie meals.

Lunch and dinner ideas

These two meal times are combined for this section simply because many of the meals are good for lunch or dinner. Pretty straightforward. These meals also try to combine protein and fiber so that you won't be too hungry. Eat of these meals are about 300 calories, and a lot of them are soup and salad! Soup is a great way to get your nutrients in an easily portioned meal. Salad is also fantastic because you can add a lot of leafy greens which are all very low-calorie vegetables. They keep you feeling full, but also provide you with essential nutrients.

- A jacket potato with salsa, sour cream, and perhaps a smidge of cheese. Cheese is delicious, so don't overdo it. Add some chives to give a bit more flavor.

- Fresh rolls with shrimp and a lot of vegetables. Vegetables that work in fresh rolls are spinach, sliced red peppers, sliced cucumbers or radishes. Use them individually or all together for some excellent flavor. Add some sauce on the side, like soy sauce or peanut sauce to dip your fresh rolls in. Avoid sauces full of sugar.

- Onion and potato pancakes with a side salad. This meal doesn't provide a lot of protein, so you can add a boiled egg to your side salad to help with that. But that's more calories.

- One baked chicken thigh with potatoes and swiss chard. Swiss chard can be bitter, so if this isn't a flavor profile you like, substitute with another cooked, leafy green. This meal is really filling and an excellent combination of protein and fiber.

- Winter squash and silken tofu soup. It sounds strange, but silken tofu is perfect for soups and smoothies. In this recipe, cook the squash first with your flavorings and broth, then blend it with tofu. You'll have a perfect protein and fiber combination.

- Pork ragu and polenta. This meal is very comforting and yet can provide you with good protein and fiber, plus a lot of flavor. Just check your portion sizes to ensure you're eating the right amount.

- Chicken and orzo soup. Add a lot of vegetables to the soup to provide you with more fiber.

- Cheese and broccoli soup. This doesn't sound low calorie, but it can be if you reduce how much fat you put into it. Use chicken or vegetable broth, skim or 1% milk, and only a few ounces of cheese. This will help keep the calories down and will also provide you with a delicious, warming soup.

Salads are also a great option for lunch or dinner. The key here is to have a lot of leafy greens and watch your extras. It's very easy to go overboard with a salad. Sometimes dressings can also be full of calories. You could make your own dressing by combining an oil with an acidic ingredient. For example, olive oil and lemon juice make a beautiful dressing. So does red wine vinegar and olive oil. Choose your dressing wisely and keep your toppings down. Adding protein and other toppings can provide you with a fuller meal, while also satisfying your taste buds. Some protein choices you can add to salad include shredded chicken, shrimp, tuna, beans, hard-boiled eggs or cooked tofu. All of this can satisfy the protein plus fiber combination which will tide you over your fast. Other toppings could be avocado, cheese, nuts, or seeds. While these are all delicious, you'll need to keep your portion sizes in check since it can easily exceed your calorie requirements. Nuts for example are very calorie dense. So, go easy with these kinds of toppings. Here are some salad ideas for your fast:

- Scallops and watercress. Watercress is a good option if you're bored with lettuce or spinach. You could also add crumbled bacon onto your salad for more flavor if you want to.

- Steak and arugula salad. Again, arugula is a good alternative to regular leafy greens in a salad. Arugula is perfect and slightly spicy, giving you a lot of flavor. For more flavor, add some shaved parmesan.

- Grilled corn and pepper salad with shrimp. This salad has no leafy greens, but you can add some to get a more filling lunch or dinner.

- Chickpea, cucumber, and tomato salad. Add some red onion for additional flavor if you want to. If the protein isn't enough for you, replace it with some shredded chicken.

- Caprese salad. This salad is basically mozzarella cheese and sliced tomatoes. Check how much mozzarella you use to make sure you don't go overboard.

Snacking ideas

Having one or two large meals in your day may not be your chosen style. In this case, you should consider snacking over the course of the day to stave off hunger. Your snacks could be large, or simply things to munch on. So long as you're not exceeding 600 calories on your fasting day, you should be okay. Make sure you that you keep a record of how many calories you're eating in your day, by tracking on an app or journal. Here are some snacking ideas for your reduced calorie days.

- Turkey slices and cheese slices. Try to keep it to two slices of deli turkey and two slices of deli cheese. Add some crackers or half a pita. Some sliced cucumbers and carrots can also go beautifully with it.

- Various colored grape tomatoes, two hard boiled eggs, and some wheat crackers. The number of crackers and type of crackers you choose depends on how many calories each is. Make sure you check carefully and eat the right amount.

- Sliced cucumbers and radishes. You can dip them in a little plain yogurt or hummus for some protein.

- Roasted carrots. They're delicious, so nothing else is really needed unless you want to add more flavor.

- A handful of nuts. Since nuts are calorie dense, keep their number low.

- Half a cup of frozen yogurt. The perfect dessert that also provides some protein.

- A package of plain popcorn. Popcorn is high in fiber and very filling. You won't need to eat a lot and 100 calories worth of popcorn will fill you up. If you want to add flavors, adjust your calorie count accordingly.

- A medley of fruits. This is just a fancy name for some sliced up fruits to munch on. Some good options are clementine segments, sliced apples, strawberries, and sliced kiwi. They're delicious together or on their own.

- A cup of watermelon. Watermelon is a great snack. It provides so much hydration, but also some key vitamins and electrolytes.

- A grapefruit cut in half. This is a perfect tart dessert. If you want to, sprinkle a little sugar on it for added sweetness.

- Low fat yogurt cup and a handful of blueberries. Yogurt can be really filling and satisfying when you're hungry. Try to avoid ones that have fruit on the bottom since they have a lot of sugar in them. Instead, get a reduced sugar variety, or even eat it plain.

- Vegetable plates. You often find these when you go to a party. Having a plate of carrots, broccoli, sliced bell peppers, and celery can be an excellent snacking option. They'll keep you full but with very few calories.

- String cheese. If cheese is what you crave the most, this can help satisfy you. String cheese isn't a lot of calories and is an excellent source of dairy and protein.

When you choose to snack, you still need to count your calories. Don't gorge until you're full just because all of these are low calorie snacks. A lot of low-calorie items add up to significant calorie gains very quickly. This can derail your goals for weekly calorie reduction. So, make sure you measure how much you eat and keep a record of it.

Warrior Diet: Paleo

The food for the warrior diet is different than the food requirements for the 5:2 method and the alternate day method. The warrior diet doesn't require any calorie reduction at all. In also doesn't really have restricted foods. However, a lot of people recommend following the paleo diet while also doing the warrior diet. Since the paleo diet is healthy, this recommendation isn't really going to harm you. Just remember to eat enough nutrients during your four-hour window to remain healthy.

The paleo diet is one based on our ancestors' lives. It

recommends eating foods that were similarly available in antiquity. So, there is a heavy emphasis on protein like seafood, eggs, and meat. It also emphasizes fruits and vegetables, nuts and seeds, and healthy fats. The paleo diet doesn't allow most grains, sugars, legumes or dairy. Afterall, these were based on heavy agriculture and processing. In general, unprocessed food is recommended over processed foods. So, if it's anything that has been processed, it should be avoided while on the paleo diet.

Since there isn't a calorie restriction when following the warrior diet, the calories will not be included, or really considered, in the foods mentioned in this section. These food options are paleo and will provide you with good nutrition. Just ensure you are getting enough variety to maintain your nutrition. So, don't eat way more protein than any other food group. Mix it up. While grains are prohibited in paleo diets, you can adapt it to fit your lifestyle better. Some people who follow paleo eat rice as their grain.

Breakfast ideas

Depending on your fasting schedule, you may not have a typical breakfast. Afterall, you might just break your fast at 6pm instead of 6am However, the meals can be the same or similar. Remember, before eating this breakfast meal, have something small a couple minutes before, just to readjust your body to eat again after a 20 hour fast. Here are some ideas for your breakfast meal:

- Egg and vegetable frittata. If you need to add oil, use coconut oil or avocado oil. Use a variety of vegetables to give you some different vitamins. You could add spinach, broccoli, and bell peppers. Or tomatoes, onions, and garlic. It will be delicious either way. Add a side of fruit, or a side salad to complete the meal.

- Bacon and eggs — a classic American breakfast. Bacon is allowed in the paleo diet and can provide needed flavor to any meal. Use the bacon fat to cook your eggs or discard the fat and cook your eggs in olive oil.

- Hard-boiled eggs with a cooked spinach and bacon salad. Since this is cooked, it's not really a salad, but it is quite delicious. Add some chives or onions for additional flavor.

If none of these appeal to you, you could always find some other recipes online. Fruits and vegetables are always a good breakfast option. A fruit salad with sunflower seeds can be a perfect break from eating eggs in the morning.

Lunch and dinner ideas

Because you only have a small eating window in the warrior diet, it's hard to really have three large meals. It's more likely that you'll have two meals, or just graze during the four hours. So, in this section lunch and dinner are combined. There will also be some recommendations for 'grazing,' or eating small bits consistently. Whichever path you choose, there are a lot of good food options following a paleo diet.

- Chicken salad and grapes. This may sound a little strange, but chicken salad is wonderful with grapes. You can even add some nuts with it for added texture. If you're eating a paleo version with grains, then having some whole-grain toast with the chicken salad.

- Egg salad. In case you're not bored with eggs, then egg salad can be a delicious meal. Add salsa or guacamole to add some flavor. A side salad can provide some additional nutrients and help you remain full.

- Burgers wrapped in lettuce or without any wrapping. Burgers are a great meal. You just can't eat the bun when following the paleo diet. However, if you want to add grains to your meal, then choose a whole wheat bread with your burger. Whether you have a bun or not, add onions, and other vegetables to your burger. If you want to add something with an amazing taste, then dry some tomatoes in the oven and add them to your burger. Dried tomatoes have an intense flavor which can add something to your meals.

- Salmon and vegetables. Grilled or fried salmon is

a great nutrient full meal. Add a side of cooked leafy greens like chard, spinach or arugula to add more nutrients. The fiber from the vegetables can help you remain full during your fasting period.

- Grilled chicken and salsa. Sliced grilled chicken and salsa served on a bed of vegetables can stand in for eating fajitas. Some vegetable options could be grilled onions and peppers, or something like asparagus.

- Steak stir-fry. This can be served with rice, if you're allowing grains as a part of your diet. Choose a steak that you can thinly slice and won't be tough when you cook it. Also slice up some vegetables for your stir fry. Zucchini, asparagus, and corn are good options. Cook it all in coconut oil. Added coconut aminos can give you nice flavor.

- Fresh rolls wrapped in rice 'paper.' This only works if you're allowing grains in your diet. But you can have Vietnamese style fresh rolls that are all wrapped in rice paper. Add some vegetables like peppers and cucumbers to the wrap and top with fish, and an avocado, then wrap it all up.

- Steak with sweet potatoes. This will be very filling. Having sweet potatoes with steak will give you a good mix of protein and fiber, without having to rely on grains. You can do the same combination with chicken and roasted potatoes or fish and potatoes. Add a side salad with arugula for a bit of spice.

If you want to eat constantly during your four hours, instead of having a large meal, then choose items that are whole and unprocessed. Here are some ideas:

- Raw fruits. Nearly any fruit is edible on the paleo diet. So, eat the ones you love the most. You should eat a lot of fruits and vegetables to give you the necessary fiber for your diet.

- Raw vegetables. Just choose the ones you like! Most vegetables are allowed on the paleo diet. Just don't eat legumes like beans and lentils.

- Nuts like pistachios, pecans, and almonds. Most

nuts are welcome in a paleo diet, but some are not. Peanuts for example are classified as a legume, so they can't be eaten on a paleo diet.

- Seeds like pumpkin seeds, sunflower seeds, and flax seeds. Seeds are a great snack. You can even turn them into a dessert. You can mix chia seeds, honey, and coconut milk for a delicious 'pudding.' The chia seeds soak up the milk and turn gelatinous, creating a nice dessert.

- Trail mix. Mix up some trail mix with seeds, nuts, and a little chocolate. Dark chocolate that is 70% cocoa is paleo and can give you that little bit of sweetness you're missing.

- Meat or Plant-based Jerky. If you like salty foods, then jerky can be a good paleo option. Just make sure you drink enough water to make up for the salt.

- Hard boiled eggs. Yes, here they are again. Eggs are excellent foods for snacking!

While on the warrior diet, you can eat paleo foods or just

follow a regular well-balanced meal. Either way, you'll only have four hours to eat all your required calories, so make sure your meals are nutritious.

Maintaining Well-Balanced Meals

When following a fast, it's important that you're getting the right nutrition, as I've mentioned several times before. If you don't want to follow a specific diet, then aim for healthy, wholesome foods. A good way of doing this is having a well-balanced meal.

Most of us have learned what a healthy meal constitutes in school. It was drilled into us during health class, possibly pointed to in biology class, and repeatedly mentioned by the school nurse. But most of us don't eat well-balanced meals. We instead eat what's convenient. With so many easy to find restaurants, food can be at our fingertips. Most of that food isn't healthy, and while it can be difficult for some Americans to find healthy foods, if you have them available to you, then choose wholesome foods, rather than fast foods.

If you have difficulty figuring out what makes a well-balanced meal, you can explore some of the resources provided by the U.S. Health Department. They even have a website dedicated to showing how to portion your meals and include all the food groups during your day. The website can offer you customizable meal plans that will give you nutritious meals and can provide other resources so that you can make the best meal decisions for your body type.

When you have a well-balanced meal, it means that you're eating a bit from at least three different food groups. The food groups are fruits, vegetables, grains, proteins, and dairy.

Fruit is...well...fruit. It's self-explanatory. While you want to eat some fruit each day, you're not going to eat as much as you do vegetables. Fruits can be high in sugar, so choose fruits that aren't as high and eat those more frequently. Try a variety of different kinds of fruit because they can each contain different vitamins and nutrients. So, pick and choose, and don't stick with the same fruit every day. Despite what they say, an apple a day doesn't keep the doctor away. Instead, mix up your fruit choices.

The vegetable family includes a lot of variety. Think pumpkins, corn, broccoli, onions, and beans. All of these are part of the vegetable group. They're also one of the largest families of food you should eat during your day. In general, at least one-third or half of your plate should be vegetables. Just like with fruit, you want to mix up your vegetables because they each provide a different type and number of vitamins. For example, yellow pumpkins can give you way more vitamin A than many other veggies. So, mix it up.

Grains are a large food group and the family consists of food produced by a grain plant. Some grain plants include wheat, bran, rye, rice, oats, and sometimes corn. All of this is then processed into other foods like bread, oatmeal, polenta, tortilla's, cereal, etc. All of these are a part of the grain food family. Grains should also be a large part of your meal. About one third of your plate will be grains. Whole grains are a better option than other types. Think whole-wheat bread vs. white bread. Choose brown rice over white rice. These types of grain contain more nutrients.

The protein family has a variety of different items in it. It can contain lean meats that are unprocessed, seafood, beans, nuts, and tofu. Some lean meats are lamb, beef, and pork. Sausages, hot dogs, and salami are considered processed and less healthy. You should eat these only in small quantities. But lean meat itself is quite healthy and you should eat about seven servings in a week. Seafood is another great choice and you should have at least two servings in your week. Seafood includes fish, shrimp, scallops, octopus, etc. Beans, nuts, and tofu are other kinds of protein. They are all plant based and are excellent alternatives to meat or seafood. You should try to have some meatless/plant-based foods during your week and beans can give you an alternative that will keep you full.

The dairy family is our last food group. It consists of animal products like milk, eggs, cheese, and yogurt. When you choose a dairy item, it should be a low-fat variety. Full fat yogurt can be very healthy and provide you with essential vitamins and probiotics. Dairy should only be a small percentage of your daily dietary consumption.

When choosing well-balanced meals, try to avoid heavily processed foods and fast foods. These can be full of sugar, carbs, and fats that aren't healthy for you. However, eating out every now and again is completely fine. Just don't make it a daily habit. Other foods like processed meats, alcohol, fatty foods, and 'junk' foods should be limited so that they do not take up a huge portion of your weekly eating.

While you fast, you want your food choices to give you the best balance of nutrients. So, following a well-balanced meal will help you maintain your weight, or even promote weight loss depending on what your diet was like before you started fasting. While you could eat all the right nutrients, you might still be sabotaging yourself with your portion sizes. So be aware of the portion size as well as the nutrients in each of your meals. Below, we'll explore some possible meal ideas that are well-balanced.

Breakfast ideas

When you break your fast, try to eat a combination of

protein and fiber to keep you full. It will also help you recover, if you decided to work out before fasting. Make sure that your keeping a record of what you eat so that you can check to see how your body responds to different foods after a long fasting period. Some people can have a negative reaction to eating certain foods after breaking their fast, so stay mindful about what you're eating and check in with yourself regularly to see if you're reacting badly to something you ate. Here are some great well-balanced breakfast ideas.

- Whole-grain English muffins with eggs, butter, and spinach. Add a side of fruit like mixed berries or a banana. This meal covers four food groups: grains, protein, dairy, and vegetables.

- Oatmeal with sunflower seeds, diced apple, and a bit of yogurt. This meal has items from four food groups. The yogurt is your protein, and the oatmeal is your fiber and grain. So, this meal will keep you fuller than just eating toast alone.

- Whole grain bread with peanut butter or a nut butter alternative. Add some fruit on the side or on the sandwich itself. Consider blueberries on top of peanut butter and toast. Or bananas. Bananas and peanut butter are magic.

- Yogurt with fruit, nuts, and some crumbled granola. This meal provides you four different food groups. This is heavier in dairy, so you would want to have less dairy in the rest of your day. Alternatively, you can substitute dairy for non-dairy milk options as well if you are dairy-intolerant. Increase how much fruit you add if you want to have a fiber rich breakfast.

- Cheese omelette with diced peppers, onions, and broccoli. Eat it with a side of toast if you want to add a grain.

A lot of the meals listed here have items from four food groups. You don't have to do that for your meals. These are just recommendations. In general, just make sure you combine a protein and fiber to keep you full. An example would be having Raisin Bran cereal (fiber) with a cup of 2% milk (protein).

Lunch ideas

With lunch, try to make a good portion of your meal vegetables. This will help you meet your daily vegetable serving and give you a good amount of nutrients and vitamins. A good option is having a salad for lunch, but this can be unwilling. So, add some protein and one other food group. All of this can help you have a satisfying lunch while fasting. Here are some lunch ideas.

- Cobb salad with a mix of leafy greens, roasted beets, tomatoes, crumbled blue cheese, and hard-boiled eggs. If you don't want to eat eggs with your lunch, substitute them for canned beans. Black beans and roasted chickpeas are good alternatives.

- Shrimp bowl with brown rice, lime flavored shrimp, sliced tomatoes, and avocado salsa. This meal provides you with your protein and fiber. It also gives you some tasty foods with avocado salsa and lime-flavored shrimp. If you're warming it up at work, check in with your coworkers, just in case the scent of seafood is off putting for anyone else around the office.

- Roasted chicken, with arugula salad and roasted new potatoes. This meal is one that you could also have for dinner. You could bring the leftovers for lunch. Whichever way, it will be filling and be a tasty alternative to eating out for lunch.

- Jacket sweet potato with corn salsa, sour cream, and black beans. This vegetarian lunch provides you with a lot of protein from the beans and sour cream. If you don't want to eat sour cream, then replace it with plain Greek yogurt.

- Five bean chilies. This will have a lot of protein and fiber from the beans, as well as a good amount of vegetables from the tomatoes, onions, and garlic in the chili.

If these don't appeal to you, then find some recipes online that look interesting. Don't feel limited by what's listed here. There are so many recipes out there that can help you choose healthy options while also being very delicious. Take some time to pick out some things you can cook and eat during the week. This will make your fasting easier if you already have your meals planned out.

Dinner ideas

This is usually your last meal before your fast. So, you want to make it very nutritious and something that will help tide you over your fasting period. If you're going to bed immediately after eating, then choose things that aren't going to disrupt your sleep. Some people feel like dairy before bed gives them nightmares, so if you're one of those people, skip dairy in your dinner. If you're having disrupted sleep but don't know the cause, then check your food journal. What did you eat before bed every night? Perhaps the problem is there. Or perhaps the problem is elsewhere. Having a record of your food choices can help you make the best decisions for your health.

To make your meal planning easier, make enough dinner to bring the extras for lunch the next day. This can help you make fasting easier. You could also plan your meals for the week on the weekends, then spend your time cooking them during your weekend. This way, all your meals are already prepared, and you just must reach into the fridge for one type to eat. Having your meals planned out will help you while you're fasting. It will also reduce and feelings of food obsession, since you'll already have things prepared and won't be constantly thinking of other foods. Here are some well-balanced meal ideas:

- Beef and cheese lasagna. Add vegetables in between the layers for added nutrients. Some great options are sliced eggplant, roasted red peppers, even some spinach. All of them can add to the value of your meal. If this doesn't appeal to you, then eat the lasagna with a side salad, using a variety of vegetables. Keep your portions small since lasagna can have a lot of cheese in it.

- Steamed trout with a side of new potatoes and swiss chard. This is one of my favorite meals. Trout is delicious and full of good antioxidants. It also tends to be less expensive than salmon, making it affordable and accessible. Swiss chard is bitter, and some people don't like it. If it's not your cup of tea, then replace it with other leafy vegetables like collard greens or kale.

- Chicken curry with potatoes and green peas. Depending on how you make your curry sauce, you should have a lot of vegetables already in the curry itself. The spices in curry are very good for you and can provide a lot of nutrients.

- Pumpkin soup with cashews and coconut milk. This is honestly divine. You'll get your protein from the coconut milk and cashews, with the fiber from the pumpkin. It's very smooth and decadent. If this flavor profile isn't for you, try it with chicken broth replacing the coconut milk, and crumbled bacon replacing the cashews. As some thyme to taste.

- Slow-cooked shredded pork tacos. Use roasted pineapple in the tacos and add thinly sliced vegetables like radishes or lettuce. Choose whole wheat or corn tortillas to wrap your tacos, and top with salsa or guacamole.

Try to have at least a couple servings of fish in your week and consider some meatless meals. Eating too much meat is not very healthy, so mix it up. Replace some meat in your favorite recipes with tofu or beans instead.

To conclude this chapter, all these different kinds of foods and meals can help you be successful with your intermittent fast. Choose the type of diet you want to follow for your fast, or don't change your diet at all. The choice is entirely up to you. If you notice that you're gaining weight while on the fast, then look at your diet. It may be the problem. If you're not satisfied with what you're currently eating on your fast, then change your diet! For people who are not following the 5:2 or alternative day method, try to maintain a diet that has at least 1,300 calories during your days. Otherwise you'll be in danger of becoming malnourished. Good luck with your meals on the fast!

Chapter 7: Motivation to Stick with Your Plan

I wish I could tell you that fasting is all sunshine and roses. I wish I could tell you that it's so easy to follow. Unfortunately, it's not. There are going to be days when you look at your cup of coffee and cry because you can't eat anything for another four hours. There are going to be days when you throw yourself at the doors of the local cafe and ogle all the pastries and lattes, knowing that by the time you can eat, the doors will be closed. There will be days when all your friends are out drinking and partying, and your eating window just ended. Basically, there are going to be frustrating days, sad days, difficult days, stressful days, and nightmare days where you're going to want to throw in the towel and give up on your fast. These are the kinds of days that you'll need motivation to help you continue your fast. Without the motivation, it's likely that you'll end your fasting period early, not start the next fasting period, or just give up all together.

One key thing you can do to keep yourself motivated is to remind yourself of the days that were amazing. Think about that day last week, when you had your latte and your boss didn't yell at you. Think about that morning, when your dogs lovingly jumped on the bed and woke you up with millions of kisses. Think about that time that you dropped your scarf on the train and someone found it and returned it to you. The recollection of these good days can help remind you that your days will get better. You can use these reminders on the rough days when you just want to give up on fasting, or the days when you just want to sit on the bathroom floor and cry.

When your days are rough and you have the stress of fasting on top of that, it's likely that you'll break your fast. However, it's important that you continue your fast again in the future, even if you hit some speed bumps along the way. This chapter will cover some points that may help you continue to feel motivated.

Distract Yourself

Sometimes the hunger that comes with fasting can be overwhelming. This is especially true with fasts that require 24 hours of not eating. If you can't seem to stop thinking about food, or if you're just feeling gnawing hunger, then you might want to break your fast early and just eat everything in front of you. Before doing that, see if some distractions will help you maintain your fasts. Some good distractions include work, exercise, and meditation.

Work probably shouldn't be classified as a distraction, but it can be a useful one when you're fasting. Having your mind occupied by something that requires you to be actively engaged is a great way to distract yourself from your feelings of hunger. Many of us have already experienced this. If you've ever been in the 'flow' while working, you've probably skipped meals without realizing it. You may have even come out of flow and realized that hours have gone by and your stomach is growling at you. This realization can help you when you're fasting. You can try to get into a state of flow, but if that is beyond you at that moment, then just get engaged with work. Start a new project or plan. If your work is very active, then get fully engaged with the activity. If your work is passive, then find another way to distract yourself.

One way of distracting yourself is to do some light exercises. Depending on the fast you're following, heavy exercise might be too much. Light exercises on the other hand, can be a great distraction and won't affect you negatively. Light exercises include things like walking and yoga. They aren't high intensity and don't involve too much effort on your part. So, they shouldn't cause you to feel nauseous or faint. Walking outside in nature is a perfect distraction. Instead of walking and focusing on your hunger, focus on things outside of you. Look at the trees, birds, and insects. Observe the other people around you, breathe in deeply, and just walk. Allow your mind to wander, but if it keeps going to your hunger, then refocus on something else. Yoga is another way that you can distract yourself. Because it requires more focus on the positions and your breath, you will quickly find yourself distracted from your hunger.

Use your distractions wisely. While it's okay to distract yourself from feeling hungry, it's not okay to distract yourself from feeling intensely uncomfortable. If you're feeling unwell, then this is a sign to step back from the fast and speak to a doctor. Don't "power through" something that isn't working for you.

Remind Yourself of Your Goals

When you fast, you usually have reasons for why you are choosing to do it. Maybe your goal is to lose weight, maybe it's just gone get healthier in general. Your goals should be personal to you, not something that's mimicry of other people's goals. Think about why you really want to fast. Think about a goal that will really motivate you to continue fasting. Whatever your reasoning, your goals can help you maintain motivation. To help you remember your goals, write them down. You can put them in the same journal you put your food notes in, or you can make a specific fasting journal with your fasting schedule, food notes, and goals all together. Having them written down makes them more concrete and gives you something to look back on when your fast becomes difficult to sustain.

As you start to feel weary of continuing your fast, or if

you struggle with the hours without food, then take the time to say your goals. Write them down somewhere so you see them frequently. You can use a dry erase marker and put your goals on your bathroom mirror. That way every day as you start your eating window you can see your goals, and every evening as you bring your eating window to a close, you're reminded of why you're fasting. During the day, when you struggle with your fast, take a moment to repeat your goals to yourself. You can say it like a mantra to help you stay focused and ignore the hunger.

Beyond repeating your goals to yourself, you can create a visual to help embody your goals. You can create a vision board. A lot of people create these boards to help remind them of their goals in many aspects of their lives. Usually, it's created with cutouts from magazines or printed pictures. Each image represents something specifically to you. If your goal is to buy a house, then you might have a picture of a beautiful house. For fasting, if your goal is to be healthier, then your picture can be anything that embodies the word 'health' to you. It could be people exercising, or even just a mountain with clean air. Your images are unique to you. Once you have your goal images, put them together in a collage and post them somewhere that you'll see your vision board every day. Your office or kitchen, maybe your bedroom, are all good choices.

Finally, if fasting is really getting you down and you don't have your vision board or written goals near at hand, then do a visualization technique. Close your eyes and in your mind, visualize yourself as you have reached your goal. What do you look like? What emotions do you feel? How do you feel physically? How do you feel mentally? Consider all these questions to help you visualize your goal achievement. This can help you remain motivated to fasting, and give you the encouragement to keep going, even after you've broken your fast.

Be Compassionate Towards Yourself

Have you ever notices that the closer we are to someone, the harsher we are to them? Like, our acquaintances see us as these perfect angels, but our friends know that we have a sharp wit, and an even sharper tongue. Our family knows that we don't take no nonsense from anyone and our family gets a big brunt of our anger when we feel miserable. But the person we treat the worst is ourselves. Any slight failure or disillusionment results in us reprimanding ourselves. Comments like, "I'm so stupid" or "Why am I such an idiot?" are things that we say to ourselves. We would never say them to our friends or acquaintances. So, we're insanely harsh to ourselves.

When to hit a snag with fasting, maybe cheat a little with what we eat or skip a fasting period, it's not uncommon for us to have some self-recriminating thoughts. These thoughts aren't beneficial. They often tear us down without providing an area to build ourselves up again. They can be extremely negative and result in us giving up our fasts all together. Instead of sulking with our own thoughts and giving up on our fasts, we should try to practice a little self-kindness.

What would you say to a friend who said they failed at their fast and they're so stupid? Would you agree with them? That's unlikely. It's more likely that you'll try to console them, reassure them that they aren't stupid, and follow up by encouraging them to continue trying. Do the same thing that you would do for a friend but do it for yourself. Instead of saying, "I'm so stupid, I failed," say, "I took a cheat day, and that's okay. I'll get right back into my fasting schedule." Be positive and compassionate towards yourself. We all make mistakes and we all have lapses. Simply learn from your experience, adapt your fasting schedule to accommodate what you've learned, and start fasting again. Don't give up just because of a little bump in the road.

Get Some Support + Bonus 16/8 method

Things are always easier with support. Some of us like to think that we're eagles, living solo among all the turkeys. We want to be free without anyone there to back us up. We don't need them! But this isn't ideal, especially when things are difficult. Sometimes, it's better to be surrounded by turkeys who care about you and will support you. Sometimes it's better to be the turkey because you know you're lovingly supported by your friends and family with you. What I'm trying to say here is that when you struggle with intermittent fasting, having the support of your friends can really make a difference in your success or failure.

If you have some friends who are very supportive of you, make sure they know when you're struggling with your fasting goals. They can probably give you a good shoulder to cry on and may even give you some tips for how to make things easier. If you're very lucky, your friends may join your fast with you. This way, you can keep each other accountable. If they don't want to fast, that's okay too so long as they're supportive of you following your health goals.

If you're truly an eagle, alone in the world, then seek support from online communities. There are a lot of blogs and forums out there, dedicated to intermittent fasting. Join some of them and talk to others who are struggling. Some great forums to join include the Reddit forum on intermittent fasting. There, they post pictures of success, questions about speed bumps, and even give each other motivation. Get involved and you'll have some support too.

To conclude this chapter, fasting is hard, but it can be done with the right support behind you and the motivation to push forward. Keep persevering, keep trying, and only give up if your body can't handle the fast. Even when you make a mistake or take a cheat day (or month), just try again when you're ready. Keep trying.

Chapter bonus: 16/8 schedule

Step 1: Planning Your Eating Schedule

This may be the biggest change that you experience as you transition from other fasting types. If you were previously doing the 14/10 method, then this won't be a huge change, but if you're transitioning from the 5:2 method or the alternate-day method, then you'll need to work on your eating schedule. You only have eight hours to eat during your day, so you need to plan when you'll have your meals. This will help ensure you don't get hangry during your day and you have enough in your system to keep you good during your fast time. Determine how you are going to break your fast and end your fast. Consider when you'll eat during the day and how that will fit into your regular schedule. Also consider how you'll handle special occasions with your friends and family.

Just like it was discussed in the transition for beginners,

consider whether you will follow this fast daily or only a couple days a week. You'll reap the most benefits from a daily fast, but it's up to you and your lifestyle.

One thing to consider when making your schedule is following your natural circadian rhythm. This was discussed in detail in chapter 1 and again in the section about transitioning from scratch, but we're mentioning it again in case you skipped that section. Following your circadian rhythm is something to keep in mind for your fasting schedule. Most people have a slump in the middle of the day, around 3:00 p.m. You have the most energy in the morning, so you want to take advantage of your natural circadian rhythm. Then you can time your eating window to start at 7:00 a.m. and end at 3:00 p.m. This will put your body in a better metabolic state and help your body burn more fat than if you eat late at night. This schedule might not work for everyone, especially if you do shift work or if you have a family you're caring for. So, find a schedule that works for you and take advantage of the times you feel naturally more energized in your day.

Finally, ensure that you are also maintaining your own

sleep schedule. You'll need to have a set sleeping time and waking time to better time your fast. If you followed the 5:2 method or alternate-day method, this might not have been so important. After all, you could eat regularly every other day, and it didn't really matter how many hours you slept. However, having a set sleep schedule will help you determine how many hours to fast while on the 16/8 method. If you sleep eight hours a night, you will only need to fast for an additional eight hours when you're awake. If you get less sleep, you'll need to adjust your fasting time during the day.

Step 2: Starting Your Transition

Your transition schedule is going to follow the same as the beginner's schedule, except you'll need to start from a day when you've done regular eating. If you're currently following the 5:2 method or the alternate-day method, make sure that you are eating enough calories the day before you start your new fast schedule. Then that night, you can start your fast. Here's the schedule, which is the same for beginners:

In week 1, for the first three days, stop eating an hour before you go to bed and start eating one hour after you wake up. This puts you at a 10-hour fast, with 14 hours to eat. After those first three days, you're going to add an hour before bed and after waking up. So, you'll stop eating two hours before bed and start eating two hours after waking up. This puts you at 12 hours of fasting and 12 hours of eating. Three days later, add another two hours, bringing you up to 14 hours of fasting and 10 hours of eating. Then finally, extend to the full 16 hours of fasting and 8 hours of eating. This schedule is perfect if you're planning on doing the midday eating window or late day eating window. But if you want to do an early morning eating window, then move your fasting hours to before bed. For instance, in the first three days, stop eating two hours before bed. Then the next three days, stop eating four hours before bed. Continue until the last three transition days, where you stop eating six or eight hours before bed.

Both transitions should slowly get you into the full fast and help curb the discomfort you might feel. This will take about two weeks to get to the full fast.

You can jump right into the 16/8 method if you were previously following the 12/12 method or the 14/10 method. You can jump right into the 16/8 from any other method, too, but you might experience some discomfort from the change.

Step 3: Preparing for Discomfort

Since you've fasted before, you probably know about the discomfort you might feel at the beginning of a new fast. If you're transitioning from a fast that included severe calorie restrictions, like the 5:2 fast, then be prepared for how eating more in a day will change your body. You might feel bloated or some gastric distress. For everyone else who has been fasting without calorie restrictions, just keep in mind that each transition brings its own level of discomfort. You might not have any issues if you're changing from the 14/10 fast to the 16/8 fast, but just be prepared in case. Keep in mind any warning signs that you should talk to a doctor about. Things like dizziness, vertigo, feeling weak, or changes in your heart rate all require you to see your doctor. If you're feeling particularly weak after shifting to the 16/8 method, then make sure that your meals have enough calories and are well-balanced.

Step 4: *Recording Things in Your Journal*

Keep a fasting journal for your 16/8 fast. If you've kept one before, then just add to it with your new fasting plan. Record your new goals, all the changes you're going through, and what you are experiencing with the change in eating schedule. Find areas where you are feeling better with the change and areas where you might be feeling discomfort. It's important to record these instances because you can then go back and determine what might be causing discomfort. Maybe it was a meal you ate or poor sleep the night before. Having a record of your day to day while fasting can help you control how your body is feeling. One thing to record is your meals. You want to make sure you're getting enough calories during the day and that you're feeling full enough that you won't be hungry in the middle of the day.

Typical **Schedule** for the 16/8 method

We've gone over the step-by-step process of transitioning into your fast. We've also looked a bit at making sure you have a clear record of the steps you are taking and how your body is adapting to the fast. Now let's look at some possible schedules for your fast. There is a schedule for your transition period and a schedule that examines what your daily eating times and windows will look like. Here are some additional things to keep in mind before looking at schedules:

- *Your choice of schedule is personal.* Create one based on your work schedule or other circumstances in your life. If you want to have dinner with your family, then use that meal to close out your eating window. Count back eight hours to figure out when your first meal will be.

- *Your fasting schedule doesn't have to be set in stone.* Try out different times or change your fasting window for special occasions. You don't want to be limited by your schedule, especially when it comes to your social life.

- A great option for scheduling is to follow the times when you're naturally more awake and aware and end your fast before your natural slumps. Each person has a different internal clock, so determine your schedule based on that. Following your natural circadian rhythm is a good place to start; adapt from there.

Early Eating Schedule

This schedule is a great option because it takes advantage of your circadian rhythm. It also is the ideal time in general to eat because it avoids eating late at night. However, it means that you're going to eat an early dinner, which might not work for everyone. With this schedule, you'll start eating at 7:00 a.m. and end at 3:00 p.m.

Here is how to ease into your fast:

Time	Days 1–3	Days 4–6	Days 7–9	Days 10–12
7:00 a.m.	Wake up Eat	Wake up Eat	Wake up Eat	Wake up Eat
9:00 a.m.				
11:00 a.m.	Eat	Eat	Eat	Eat
1:00 p.m.				
3:00 p.m.	Snack		Eat	Eat before 3
5:00 p.m.		Eat	Fast	Fast
7:00	Eat	Fast	Fast	Fast

p.m.				
9:00 p.m.	Fast	Fast	Fast	Fast
10:00 p.m.	Sleep/fast	Sleep/fast	Sleep/fast	Sleep/fast

Here is your weeklong schedule once you've eased into the fast:

Time	12:00 a.m.– 7:00 a.m.	7:00 a.m.	11:00 a.m.	2:00 p.m.	3:00 p.m.– 2:00 a.m.
Monday to Sunday	Fast/sleep	Breakfast (either light or the	Large meal	Last meal, finished by 3:00	Fast/sleep

		largest meal of the day)		p.m.	

Midday Eating Schedule

Some people have difficulty with eating first thing in the morning. In this case, you can start your fast later in the day. This fast is ideal for people who want to eat right in the middle of the day. It gives you time to wind down before bed and prepare your body for a time of rest without too much digestion happening while you sleep. It also gives you time to exercise in the morning before you break your fast if you want to.

Here is how to ease into your fast:

Time	Days 1–3	Days 4–6	Days 7–9	Days 10–12

6:00 a.m.	Sleep/eat	Sleep/east	Sleep/fast	Sleep/fast
8:00 a.m.	Eat	Eat	Eat	Fast
10:00 a.m.				Eat
12:00 p.m.	Eat	Eat	Eat	
2:00 p.m.	Snack	Snack		Eat
4:00 p.m.				
6:00 p.m.	Eat	Eat	Eat	Eat before 6:00 p.m.

8:00 p.m.			Fast	Fast
10:00 p.m.	Sleep/fast	Sleep/fast	Sleep/fast	Sleep/fast

Here is your weeklong schedule once you've eased into the fast:

Time	12:00 a.m.– 7:00 a.m.	10:00 a.m.	2:00 p.m.	5:00 p.m.	6:00 p.m.– 12:00 a.m.
Monda	Fast/sle	Breakfa	Larg	Last	Fast/sle

y to Sunday	ep	st (either light or the largest meal of the day)	e meal	meal, finished by 6:00 p.m.	ep

Evening Eating Schedule

This schedule doesn't take advantage of your circadian rhythm, and it might not give you the most benefits in changing glucose and cortisol levels. However, this schedule can work for people who really appreciate social eating or people who work at unconventional hours. You can always eat a bit earlier to change this schedule.

Here is how to ease into your fast:

Time	Days 1–3	Days 4–6	Days 7–9	Days 10–12
12:00 a.m.–6:00 a.m.	Sleep/fast	Sleep/fast	Sleep/fast	Sleep/fast
8:00 a.m.	Fast	Fast	Fast	Fast
10:00 a.m.	Eat	Fast	Fast	Fast
12:00 p.m.		Eat	Fast	Fast
2:00 p.m.	Eat		Eat	Fast
4:00 p.m.	Snack	Eat	Snack	Eat

6:00 p.m.		Snack		
8:00 p.m.	Eat		Eat	Eat
10:00 p.m.		Eat		
12:00 a.m.			Eat	Eat before midnight

Here is your week-long schedule once you've eased into the fast:

Time	12:00	8:00	4:00	8:00	11:00

	a.m.–8:00 a.m.	a.m.–4:00 p.m.	p.m.	p.m.	p.m.–12:00 a.m.
Monday to Sunday	Fast/sleep	Fast	Breakfast (either light or the largest meal of the day)	Large meal	Last meal, finished by midnight

These three different schedules give you some options for following your 16/8 fasting schedule. As mentioned before, adapt the schedules to better fit your own daily rhythm and lifestyle. It's ideal if your schedule is consistent, but it doesn't have to be set in stone. If you know you want to celebrate your best friend's promotion at the end of the week, then shift your fasting schedule to accommodate eating with your friends. Remember, fasting isn't a diet; it's just an eating schedule. It doesn't need to be permanent, and there shouldn't be any guilt about shifting your schedule. Since we've now discussed several schedule possibilities and how to ease into them, we'll spend the next couple of chapters looking at food choices and some meal plans.

Conclusion

Well look at that! You've made it to the end of the book. I hope the journey was worth it and that you're now ready to start your intermittent fasting schedule. We've covered many topics within these chapters. You now know the basics of intermittent fasting. You know what it is, and the different types of fasts. You know the myths associated with fasting and the benefits and risks of starting a fast. You know exactly how to transition into your fast and what foods will give you the most advantages while fasting. You also know ways to help you stay motivated.

Intermittent fasting is a great way to take control of your health and weight. I would wholeheartedly recommend it to anyone who is struggling to change their relationship with food. Therefore, I wrote this book! I hope the book has helped you learn more about fasting and I also hope you'll give it a chance. Remember to take it slow and really consider all aspects of fasting before diving in. It's a great opportunity to improve your life so hopefully you'll try it. Good luck with your health and wellness journey!

References

The Editors of Encyclopedia Britannica. (n.d.). Fasting. Retrieved from https://www.britannica.com/topic/fasting

Alhamdan, B. A., Garcia-Alvarez, A., Alzahrnai, A. H., Karanxha, J., Stretchberry, D. R., Contrera, K. J., ... Cheskin, L. J. (2016). Alternate day versus daily energy restriction diets: which is more effective for weight loss? A systematic review and meta-analysis. Obesity Science & Practice, 2(3), 293–302. doi: 10.1002/osp4.52

Anson, R. M., Guo, Z., Cabo, R. D., Iyun, T., Rios, M., Hagepanos, A., ... Mattson, M. P. (2003). Intermittent fasting dissociates beneficial effects of dietary restriction on glucose metabolism and neuronal resistance to injury from calorie intake. Proceedings of the National Academy of Sciences, 100(10), 6216–6220. doi: 10.1073/pnas.1035720100

Azevedo, F. R. D., Ikeoka, D., & Caramelli, B. (2013). Effects of intermittent fasting on metabolism in men. Revista Da Associação Médica Brasileira, 59(2), 167–

173. doi: 10.1016/j.ramb.2012.09.003

Berg, J. M., Stryer, L., Tymoczko, J. L., & Gatto, G. J. (2019). Biochemistry. New York: Macmillan international higher education.

Bjarnadottir, A. (2016, October 12). Alternate-Day Fasting - A Comprehensive Beginner's Guide. Retrieved from https://www.healthline.com/nutrition/alternate-day-fasting-guide#section1

Cox, O. (2015). The Five Food Groups. Retrieved from https://www.eatforhealth.gov.au/food-essentials/five-food-groups

Furmli, S., Elmasry, R., Ramos, M., & Fung, J. (2018). Therapeutic use of intermittent fasting for people with type 2 diabetes as an alternative to insulin. BMJ Case Reports. doi: 10.1136/bcr-2017-221854

Gunnars, K. (2018). The Paleo Diet - A Beginner's Guide Meal Plan. Retrieved from https://www.healthline.com/nutrition/paleo-diet-meal-plan-and-menu#section8

Gunnars, K. (2019, July 22). 11 Myths About Fasting and

Meal Frequency. Retrieved from https://www.healthline.com/nutrition/11-myths-fasting-and-meal-frequency#section11

Heilbronn, L. K., Smith, S. R., Martin, C. K., Anton, S. D., & Ravussin, E. (2005). Alternate day fasting in nonobese subjects: effects on body weight, body composition, and energy metabolism. The American Journal of Clinical Nutrition, 81(1), 69–73. doi: 10.1093/ajcn/81.1.69

Keys, A., Brozek, J., Henshel, A., Mickelson, O., & Taylor, H. L. (1950). The biology of human starvation (Vol. 1-2). Minneapolis, MN: University of Minnesota Press.

Klempel, M. C., Bhutani, S., Fitzgibbon, M., Freels, S., & Varady, K. A. (2010). Dietary and physical activity adaptations to alternate day modified fasting: implications for optimal weight loss. Nutrition Journal, 9(1). doi: 10.1186/1475-2891-9-35

Klempel, M. C., Kroeger, C. M., Bhutani, S., Trepanowski, J. F., & Varady, K. A. (2012). Intermittent fasting combined with calorie restriction is effective for weight loss and cardio-protection in obese women. Nutrition Journal, 11(1). doi: 10.1186/1475-2891-11-98

Kubala, J. (2018). The Warrior Diet: Review and Beginner's Guide. Retrieved from https://www.healthline.com/nutrition/warrior-diet-guide#benefits

Martin, B., Mattson, M. P., & Maudsley, S. (2006). Caloric restriction and intermittent fasting: Two potential diets for successful brain aging. Ageing Research Reviews, 5(3), 332–353. doi: 10.1016/j.arr.2006.04.002

Patterson, R. E., Laughlin, G. A., Lacroix, A. Z., Hartman, S. J., Natarajan, L., Senger, C. M., ... Gallo, L. C. (2015). Intermittent Fasting and Human Metabolic Health. Journal of the Academy of Nutrition and Dietetics, 115(8), 1203–1212. doi: 10.1016/j.jand.2015.02.018

(n.d.). Prediabetes - Your Chance to Prevent Type 2 Diabetes | CDC. Retrieved from https://www.cdc.gov/diabetes/basics/prediabetes.html

Schübel, R., Nattenmüller, J., Sookthai, D., Nonnenmacher, T., Graf, M. E., Riedl, L., ... Kühn, T. (2018). Effects of intermittent and continuous calorie restriction on body weight and metabolism over 50 wk: a randomized controlled trial. The American Journal of Clinical Nutrition, 108(5), 933–945. doi: 10.1093/ajcn/nqy196

Wolff, C. (n.d.). 7 Things Nutritionists Wish You Knew About the Warrior Diet. Retrieved from https://www.rd.com/health/diet-weight-loss/warrior-diet/

CPSIA information can be obtained
at www.ICGtesting.com
Printed in the USA
BVHW080025190521
607637BV00004B/429